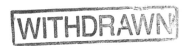

Baillière's
CLINICAL
PAEDIATRICS

INTERNATIONAL PRACTICE AND RESEARCH

Baillière's

CLINICAL
PAEDIATRICS

INTERNATIONAL PRACTICE AND RESEARCH

Volume 4/Number 2
May 1996

Paediatric Endocrinology

CHRISTOPHER J. H. KELNAR MA, MD, FRCP, DCH
Guest Editor

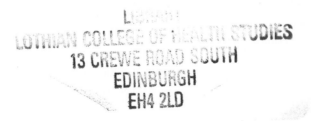

Baillière Tindall
London Philadelphia Sydney Tokyo Toronto

This book is printed on acid-free paper.

Baillière Tindall   24–28 Oval Road
W.B. Saunders   London NW1 7DX, UK
Company Ltd
             The Curtis Center, Independence Square West,
             Philadelphia, PA 19106–3399, USA

             55 Horner Avenue
             Toronto, Ontario M8Z 4X6, Canada

             Harcourt Brace & Company
             Australia
             30–52 Smidmore Street, Marrickville, NSW 2204, Australia

             Harcourt Brace & Company
             Japan Inc
             Ichibancho Central Building,
             22–1 Ichibancho, Chiyoda-ku, Tokyo 102, Japan

Whilst great care has been taken to maintain the accuracy of the information contained in this issue, the authors, editor, owners and publishers cannot accept any responsibility for any loss or damage arising from actions or decisions based on information contained in this publication; ultimate responsibility for the treatment of patients and interpretation of published material lies with the medical practitioner. The opinions expressed are those of the authors and the inclusion in this publication of material relating to a particular product, method or technique does not amount to an endorsement of its value or quality, or of the claims made by its manufacturer.

ISSN 0963–6714

ISBN 0–7020–2180–6 (single copy)

Baillière's Clinical Paediatrics is published four times each year by Baillière Tindall. Prices for Volume 4 (1996) are:

TERRITORY	ANNUAL SUBSCRIPTION	SINGLE ISSUE
Europe including UK	£90.00 (Institutional) post free £50.00 (Individual) post free	£30.00 post free
All other countries	Consult your local Harcourt Brace & Company office	

The editor of this publication is Gail Greensmith, Baillière Tindall, 24–28 Oval Road, London NW1 7DX, UK.

Baillière's Clinical Paediatrics is covered in Index Medicus, Current Contents/Clinical Medicine, Current Contents/Life Sciences, the Science Citation Index, SciSearch, Research Alert and Excerpta Medica.

Baillière's Clinical Paediatrics was published from 1972 to 1986 as *Clinics in Paediatrics*

Typeset by Phoenix Photosetting, Chatham.
Printed and bound in Great Britain by the University Printing House, Cambridge, UK.

Contributors to this issue

TIM D. CHEETHAM BSc, MBChB, MRCP, Clinical Lecturer, Department of Paediatrics, Addenbrooke's Hospital, Level 8, Hills Road, Cambridge CB2 2QQ, UK.

PAUL CZERNICHOW MD, Professor, Head of the Pediatric and Diabetology Unit, Hôpital Robert Debré, 48 boulevard Sérurier, 75019 Paris; Professor of Pediatrics, Faculte Saint Louis Lariboisiere, France.

ANNETTE GRÜTERS PD, MD, Pediatric Endocrinology, University Children's Hospital, Virchow Klinikum, Humbolt University, Heubnerweg 6, D-14059 Berlin, Germany.

SARAH J. HOLMES MA, MBBS, MRCP, Research Fellow, Department of Endocrinology, Christie Hospital, Wilmslow Road, Manchester M20 4BX, UK.

IEUAN A. HUGHES MA, MD, FRCP, FRCP(C), Professor, Department of Paediatrics, Addenbrooke's Hospital, Level 8, Hills Road, Cambridge CB2 2QQ, UK.

CHRISTIAN JUX MD, Research Fellow, University Children's Hospital, Im Neuenheimer Feld 150, D-69120 Heidelberg, Germany.

CHRISTOPHER J. H. KELNAR MA, MD, FRCP, DCH, Consultant Paediatric Endocrinologist and Senior Lecturer in Child Health, Department of Child Life and Health, University of Edinburgh, 20 Sylvan Place, Edinburgh EH9 1UW, UK.

JEAN MARC LOBACCARO PhD, INSERM U439, 70 rue de Navacelles, F-34049 Montpellier, France.

SERGE LUMBROSO MD, PhD, Unité BEDR, Hôpital Lapeyroine, F-34295 Montpellier, France.

OTTO MEHLS Professor of Pediatrics, Head, Division of Pediatric Nephrology, University Children's Hospital, Im Neuenheimer Feld 150, D-69120 Heidelberg, Germany.

NICOLAS POUJOL PhD, Unité BEDR, Hôpital Lapeyroine, F-34295 Montpellier, France.

ASAD RAHIM MBChB, MRCP, Research Fellow, Department of Endocrinology, Christie Hospital, Wilmslow Road, Manchester M20 4BX, UK.

MICHAEL B. RANKE MD, FRCP, Professor, Section of Pediatric Endocrinology, Children's Hospital, University of Tübingen, D 72070 Tübingen, Germany.

STEPHEN M. SHALET BSc, MD, FRCP, Professor of Endocrinology, Christie Hospital, Wilmslow Road, Manchester M20 4BX, UK.

CHARLES SULTAN MD, PhD, Professor of Developmental and Reproductive Biology, School of Medicine of Montpellier; Chief Paediatric Endocrinology Unit, Hôpital A. de Villeneuve, F-34295 Montpellier, France.

BURKHARD TÖNSHOFF PD, MD, Division of Paediatric Nephrology, Children's Hospital, Im Neuenheimer Feld 150, D-69120 Heidelberg, Germany.

HAMISH WALLACE MD, FRCP, Consultant Paediatric Oncologist, Royal Hospital for Sick Children, Sciennes Road, Edinburgh EH9 1LF, UK.

Table of contents

PREVIOUS ISSUES

Vol. 2, No. 1 1994
Coma
J. A. Eyre

Vol. 2, No. 2 1994
Current Issues in the Adolescent Patient
R. S. Tonkin

Vol. 2, No. 3 1994
Epilepsy
E. M. Ross & R. C. Woody

Vol. 2, No. 4 1994
Paediatric Gastroenterology
B. S. Kirschner & J. A. Walker-Smith

Vol. 3, No. 1 1995
Pulmonary Problems in the Perinatal Period and their Sequelae
V. Y. H. Yu

Vol. 3, No. 2 1995
Asthma
P. D. Phelan

Vol. 3, No. 3 1995
Stress and Pain in Infancy and Childhood
A. Aynsley-Green, M. P. Ward Platt & A. R. Lloyd-Thomas

Vol. 3, No. 4 1995
Leukaemia and Lymphoma
J. M. Chessells & I. M. Hann

Vol. 4, No. 1 1996
Cardiology for General Paediatricians
B. W. McCrindle

FORTHCOMING ISSUE

Vol. 4, No. 3 1996
Diagnosis and Management of Neurological Disabilities in Childhood
L. Rosenbloom

Preface

The optimal management of many common paediatric endocrine conditions remains controversial. Nevertheless, basic scientific advances are impinging significantly on our understanding. In addition, fetal and childhood growth may have important implications, not only in childhood but for adult health and disease. This issue describes some of these exciting developments and addresses practical treatment issues. Topics reviewed are

- intersex—the relevance of molecular genetic advances to understanding pathophysiology and practical management issues
- the implications of fetal growth failure for later dysfunction
- the effectiveness world-wide of screening programmes for congenital hypothyroidism and long-term neurodevelopmental outcomes
- management of congenital adrenal hyperplasia including the place for antenatal diagnosis and treatment, neonatal screening and morbidity outcomes
- Turner syndrome—diagnosis, associated abnormalities, optimal management of growth and puberty
- the practical implications of steroid therapy in chronic paediatric diseases—inhaled/systemic steroids in asthma, topical steroids in eczema, systemic steroids in renal disease and juvenile chronic arthritis and the pathophysiology of glucocorticoid/growth hormone axis interactions
- growth and endocrine (thyroid, adrenal, puberty) dysfunction following chemotherapy for childhood cancers
- the importance of adequate bone mineralization and relevance of the timing of puberty in prevention of adult disease

I hope that the topics covered will not only provide up to date information about important aspects of clinical paediatric practice but also stimulate thought about areas of change and controversy.

I am grateful to all the contributors and to Gail Greensmith and Karen Grace of Baillière Tindall for their expert assistance.

CHRISTOPHER J. H. KELNAR

1

Disorders of sexual differentiation: recent molecular and clinical advances

CHARLES SULTAN
JEAN MARC LOBACCARO
SERGE LUMBROSO
NICOLAS POUJOL

The various processes involved in sexual differentiation have been considerably clarified over the past few years through advances in biochemistry and molecular genetics. The cloning of the gene responsible for testicular determination (*SRY*), the anti-Müllerian hormone gene and its receptor, the aromatase gene, the genes involved in testosterone synthesis (StAR, 3β-HSD, 17β-HSD, 17α-hydroxylase,), the androgen receptor gene and the 5α-reductase gene has greatly improved our understanding of the gene defects causing abnormal sexual differentiation (Sultan et al, 1995).

From a physiological, chronological and clinical point of view, sexual differentiation includes both sexual determination, which is, for the male, the transformation of the undifferentiated gonad to a testis, and sexual differentiation, which is dependent on secretions from the fetal testis.

Sexual ambiguity can be a difficult and sometimes confusing diagnostic problem in children, resulting from discordance between the karyotype and the phenotype. Molecular analyses, including the Southern blot, mRNA expression and enzymatic amplification (PCR), along with different point mutation detecting methods and sequencing, can be used for direct diagnosis of male and female pseudohermaphroditisms.

ABNORMALITIES OF SEX DETERMINATION

The signal event in the male pathway, which is the differentiation of a bi-potential gonad into a testis, is regulated (in early embryogenesis) by the testis-determining factor (TDF) on the Y chromosome (Figure 1). A regulatory gene was mapped to the short arm of the Y chromosome by molecular analysis of human sex reversal (XX male and XY female) (Palmer et al, 1989; Sinclair et al, 1990). Various data, such as the finding of *de novo* mutated *SRY* gene in XY female (Berta et al, 1990) and the production of reversed XX mice after *SRY* transgenesis (Koopman et al, 1991) further confirmed that *SRY* is

Baillière's Clinical Paediatrics —
Vol. 4, No. 2, May 1996
ISBN 0–7020–2180–6
0963–6714/96/020221 + 23 $12.00/00

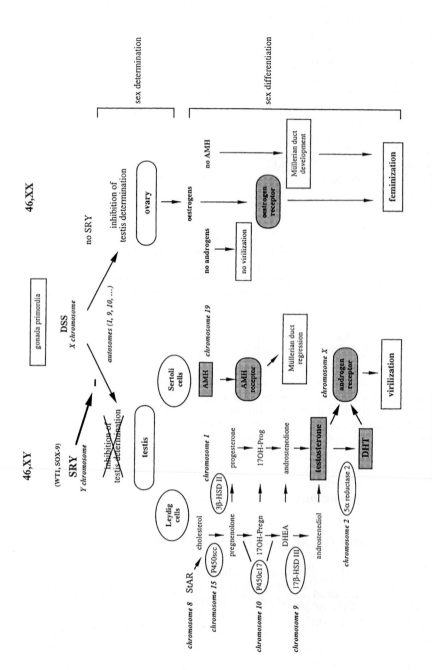

identical to TDF. This single exon gene is composed of an open reading frame of 669 bp. It encodes for a DNA binding protein that is conserved among mammalian Y chromosomes and is similar to members of the HMG box family of transcription factors. The *SRY* gene product recognizes sequence-specific sites, and the DNA binding is essential for testis determination (Hawkins, 1993). In contrast to the testis, ovary development is classically considered to be a passive process, resulting from the absence of *SRY* gene. Nevertheless, several lines of evidence suggest that *DAX-1*, the gene for X-linked congenital adrenal hypoplasia, is required for ovarian development.

Several situations resulting in abnormal testis or ovary determination can be observed (Table 1).

Table 1. Classification of sexual differentiation abnormalities.

Sex determination	Sex differentiation
Testis	*Male pseudohermaphroditism*
Defect of testis development	Persistent Müllerian duct syndrome
XY gonadal dysgenesis	Testosterone synthesis defect
—Y-linked	StAR, congenital lipoid adrenal hyperplasia
—X-linked	17α-Hydroxylase deficiency
—autosome-linked	3β-Hydroxysteroid dehydrogenase deficiency
True hermaphroditism	17β-Hydroxysteroid dehydrogenase deficiency
XX males	Androgen resistance
Klinefelter's syndrome	5α-reductase deficiency
Leydig cell hypoplasia	Androgen insensitivity syndrome
Defect of testis maintenance	
Embryonic testicular regression	*Female pseudohermaphroditism*
Rudimentary testis syndrome	Testosterone synthesis excess
Congenital anorchia	21-Hydroxylase deficiency
	11β-Hydroxylase deficiency
Ovary	3β-Hydroxysteroid dehydrogenase deficiency
Defect of ovary development	Oestrogen synthesis defect
XX gonadal dysgenesis	Aromatase deficiency
Defect of ovary maintenance	
Turner syndrome	

Testis

Defects of testis development

XY gonadal dysgenesis

Y-LINKED XY GONADAL DYSGENESIS. The syndrome of pure gonadal dysgenesis—*46,XY complete gonadal dysgenesis (Swyer syndrome)*—is characterized by the presence of bilateral streak gonads in a phenotypic female with sexual infantilism and an XY karyotype. Most individuals come to medical attention in their mid-teens or later for evaluation of problems related to lack of ovarian function.

Most of the patients do not present with sex chromosome structural abnormalities, but some sporadic cases with a deletion in the short arm of the Y chromosome or with a duplication of the short arm of the X chromosome resulting from translocation of an extra fragment of Xp on an otherwise normal Y chromosome have been noted. Gene abnormalities of *SRY*, such as deletion and point mutations, have been described in only

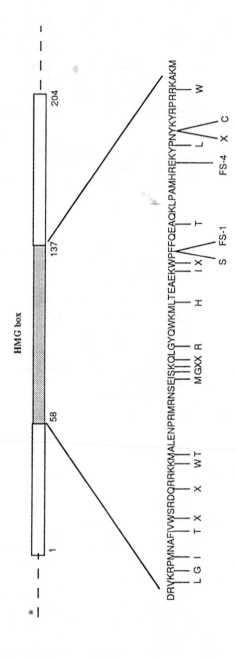

Figure 2. Sex-reversing mutations in the *SRY* gene. X indicates termination codon and FS indicates frameshift mutation. The number (n) of deleted base pairs causing frameshift is indicated as FS-n. * A large deletion outside the *SRY* gene has also been reported.

10–15% of the patients; the majority of the point mutations are located in the HMG box (Figure 2).

The management of patients with pure gonadal dysgenesis is similar to that of patients with Turner syndrome in that long-term oestrogen therapy should ideally be instituted at the expected time of puberty. Neoplastic transformation of the dysgenetic gonads is likely to occur in patients with XY pure gonadal dysgenesis, making routine gonadectomy in these patients mandatory.

Mixed gonadal dysgenesis is characterized by a unilateral testis (often intra-abdominal), a contralateral streak gonad and persistent Müllerian duct structures; it is associated with varying degrees of inadequate masculinization. The most common karyotype is 45,XO/46,XY, but other mosaics have been reported with a structurally abnormal or normal Y chromosome.

Patients with mixed gonadal dysgenesis are at increased risk of gonadal (and Wilms') tumour. It is recommended that patients with mixed gonadal dysgenesis be reared as females. This allows for removal of the gonads and the avoidance of their malignant potential. As males, patients would be infertile.

Dysgenetic male pseudohermaphroditism encompasses a large clinical heterogeneity and refers to a group of patients presenting with bilateral dysgenetic testes, persistent Müllerian structures, cryptorchidism and inadequate virilization. Because the uterus is present, the sex of rearing is female, and gonadectomy, as for mixed gonadal dysgenesis, is recommended. These patients should be routinely screened for tumour.

X-LINKED 46,XY GONADAL DYSGENESIS. Sex reversal in 46,XY patients with a duplication of the short arm of the X chromosome suggested the existence of a gene in the X chromosome, *DSS* (dosage-sensitive sex reversal), which when present in two copies could override the effect of the Y chromosome (Bardoni et al, 1994). In the 160 kb stretch within the Xp21 region containing the *DSS* locus and also the locus for adrenal hypoplasia congenita (AHC), the first, and unique, gene isolated is *DAX-1* (for the first gene in the DSS–AHC critical region of the X chromosome). *DAX-1* encodes a nuclear receptor related to steroidogenic factor 1, which has been shown in homozygous knock-out mouse to result in the absence of gonads in both sexes. The close embryological relationship between adrenals and gonads, and their shared steroidogenic properties, supports the hypothesis that *DAX-1* might be both the *DSS* and the gene responsible for AHC. In fact, mutations of *DAX-1* (Muscatelli et al, 1994) do not affect testis development, and no mutation has been described in XY females.

Although it has not been determined whether *DAX-1* is *DSS*, some information is available. Large deletions that completely remove the DSS–AHC critical region are compatible with testis development, so *DSS* must not be required in males; however, the presence of two copies results in a failure of testis development in XY individuals, so *DSS* must be repressed in order to allow male sex differentiation (see Figure 1). It thus appears that *DSS* interacts in a dose-dependent fashion with an *SRY*-related gene.

AUTOSOMAL-LINKED 46,XY GONADAL DYSGENESIS. Another gene has been isolated which also appears to exert its effects on sex determination in a dose-sensitive fashion. This gene, *SOX-9* (*SRY* box-related sequence), maps to the locus on chromosome 17, SRA1, which is associated with campomelic dysplasia and sometimes gonadal dysgenesis. *SOX-9* belongs to the same family of HMG proteins as *SRY*. Despite similarities, it does not seem that *SOX-9* and *SRY* compete with each other on a target site because it is a reduction of *SOX-9* expression (Wagner et al, 1994) that leads to sex reversal from male to female.

Several other cytogenetic abnormalities indicate and map other genes involved in the sex determination pathway; for example the monosomy of chromosomes 1, 8, 9p and 10q has been associated with sex reversal.

True hermaphroditism. True hermaphroditism is defined as the simultaneous presence of testicular and ovarian tissue in a single individual in either the same or opposite gonads. Both the external genitalia and internal duct structures of true hermaphrodites display gradations between male and female. The initial manifestations are ambiguous genitalia in 90% of cases; more rarely, isolated clitoromegaly or penile hypospadias is first noted. Two-thirds of true hermaphrodites are raised as males. Among those raised as females, two-thirds will have clitoromegaly. Virtually all patients have a urogenital sinus, and in most cases a uterus is present.

The most common peripheral karyotype is 46,XX, but mosaicisms are observed (XX, XY). The *SRY* gene is present in 10–30% of patients, suggesting that true hermaphroditism is a heterogeneous condition in terms of its genetic background.

The most important aspect of management of true hermaphrodites is gender assignment. Such decisions should be based upon the adequacy of the phallus and the findings at laparotomy. True hermaphrodites have the potential for fertility.

XX males. These patients with no genital ambiguity develop gynaecomastia at puberty. Although they present, as do patients with Klinefelter's syndrome, with some degree of testosterone deficiency and impairment of spermatogenesis, they differ from the latter in that they are not tall and show no impairment of intelligence. The *SRY* gene is present in some of the XX males, whereas others have no demonstrable Y sequences. Management of XX males is comparable to that of Klinefelter's syndrome patients.

Klinefelter's syndrome. Klinefelter's syndrome represents the most common major abnormality of sexual determination. The main characteristics of this syndrome are seminiferous tubular dysgenesis, small testes, androgenic deficiency, pubertal gynaecomastia, eunuchoidism, tall stature, intellectual impairment and psychiatric disorders. Management options for patients with Klinefelter's syndrome are limited to careful androgen supplementation in adolescence in order to improve their body image and to reduce the risk of psychiatric disorders.

Leydig cell hypoplasia. Leydig cell hypoplasia is a form of pseudohermaphroditism in which Leydig cell differentiation and testosterone production are impaired. The phenotype is female, although Müllerian structures are absent. A mutation in the sixth transmembrane domain of the LH receptor, which inhibits its function, has recently been reported in Leydig cell hypoplasia patients (Kremer et al, 1995).

Defect of testis maintenance

Bilateral vanishing testis (or embryonic testicular regression) is character-ized in patients by an XY karyotype and absent or rudimentary testes

The syndrome encompasses the presence of testes that vanish during embryogenesis. The aetiology of this syndrome is unclear: it is possible that regression of the testes in utero is due to a genetic mutation, a teratogen factor or a bilateral torsion. Clinically, the syndrome encompasses a spectrum of phenotypes, ranging in severity from genital ambiguity to a male phenotype with an empty scrotum. The management of patients with a defect of testis maintenance is dictated by their position in the clinical spectrum of the disorder.

In *true agonadism*, external genitalia are ambiguous and Müllerian derivatives absent or rudimentary owing to complete or partial anti-Müllerian hormone secretion, without secretion of testosterone.

Patients with a *rudimentary testis* have a male phenotype with micropenis and small atrophic testes with pre-Sertoli and Leydig cells. Some patients present with perineal hypospadias and persistent Müllerian derivatives.

Congenital anorchia is characterized by the complete absence of testicular tissue at birth but normal male sexual differentiation without Müllerian derivatives.

Phenotypic males require long-term androgen replacement, beginning at the time of expected puberty. Patients with ambiguous genitalia require indi-vidual assessment to determine the optimal sex of rearing. In the absence of palpable gonads, basal or hCG-stimulated testosterone secretion to a level above the female range is of interest, although laparotomy or cœlioscopy and gonadal histology are essential. Sex of rearing is male with testosterone replacement therapy, leading to a normal puberty and sexual life.

Ovary

Defect of ovary development: XX gonadal dysgenesis

Pure XX gonadal dysgenesis is characterized by a female phenotype, sexual infantilism and bilateral streak gonads. Familial cases can occur, with variable clinical expression including precocious menopause. To date, no X-linked gene mutation has been reported. Management of XX pure gonadal dysgenesis is very similar to that of Turner syndrome.

Defect of ovary maintenance: Turner syndrome

Patients with Turner syndrome have bilateral streak gonads, sexual infantilism, short stature and other somatic abnormalities. It has been demonstrated that puberty can be induced by the administration of oestrogen at the appropriate time and that the use of biosynthetic GH may accelerate long-term growth in patients with this syndrome (see Chapter 5 in this volume). Due to the increased risk of gonadoblastoma in Turner syndrome with Y material, screening for Y genes should be carried out systematically: a thorough attempt should be made to rule out occult mosaicism in these patients.

ABNORMALITIES OF SEX DIFFERENTIATION

After sex determination, the events of male sex differentiation take two pathways (Sultan et al, 1995): one inhibitory, the regression of the Müllerian ducts by action of the anti-Müllerian hormone, and the other stimulatory, which requires the two androgens testosterone and 5α-dihydrotestosterone (DHT) and a functional androgen receptor very early during embryogenesis. It has been clearly demonstrated that androgens are essential for the virilization of Wolffian duct structures, the urogenital sinus and the genital tubercule. In the urogenital sinus and the genital tubercule, testerone is converted to DHT by 5α-reductase. Testosterone or DHT then binds to a nuclear receptor to stimulate protein synthesis.

Molecular cloning and genetic, biochemical and pharmacological approaches have provided strong support for the existence of at least two steroid 5α-reductase enzymes in humans (designated as types 1 and 2 to reflect the chronological order in which the genes were isolated) (Wilson et al, 1993). Molecular genetic evidence, such as gene deletions and point mutations, has demonstrated that the 5α-reductase 2 gene is the morbid locus for 5α-reductase deficiency (Wilson et al, 1993).

The androgen receptor belongs to the subfamily of steroid hormone receptors within a larger family of nuclear proteins that activate target gene transcription through the same hormone response elements. As a member of the nuclear receptor family (Figure 3), the androgen receptor contains an N-terminal region, which is variable in length and has a role in transcriptional activation, a central cysteine-rich DNA-binding domain and a carboxy-terminal ligand-binding domain (Brinkmann, 1994).

Although the two physiologically active androgens, testosterone and DHT, interact directly with the androgen receptor and mediate hormonal responses, conversion of testosterone to the more potent agonist DHT is required in certain tissues for the androgen action to occur. This requirement is particularly clear during male sexual development, when formation of DHT is mandatory for the virilization of external genitalia and the development of the prostate gland. Virilization of the Wolffian duct structures is, however, thought to be mediated by testosterone. The actions of androgens on target cells occur via the classical steroid receptor pathway (Figure 4) (Brinkmann, 1994). After the binding of androgen to the receptor, a hyperphosphorylation, whose role is unknown, of the N-terminal domain of the protein is observed. The complex androgen-activated androgen receptor is thus able to migrate in the nucleus and

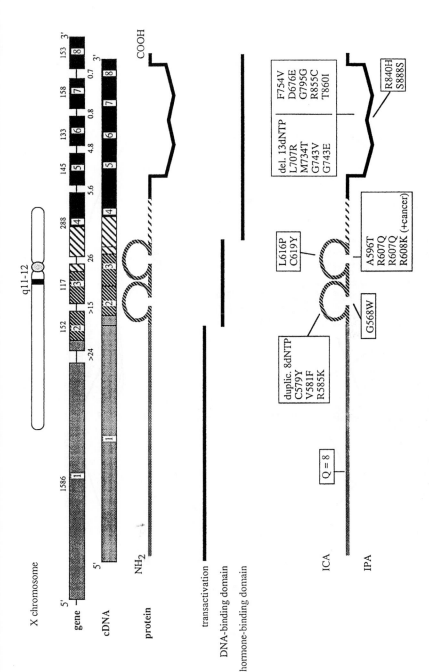

Figure 3. Top: Schematic representation of the androgen receptor gene and protein organization. Bottom: Androgen receptor abnormalities (personal data). The single amino acid letter code is used.

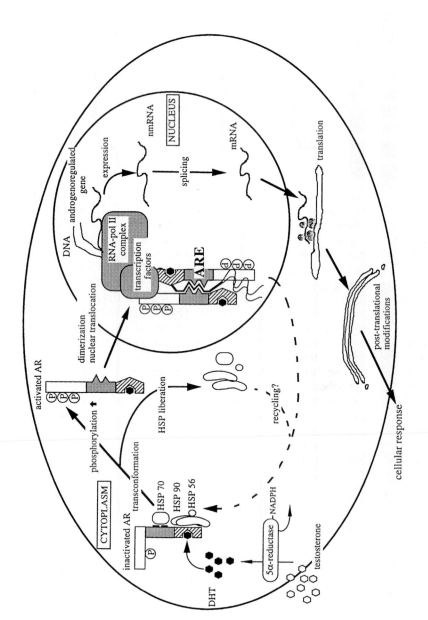

Figure 4. Schematic representation of the androgen action in target cell. HSP = heat shock protein; ARE = androgen response element.

interact as a homodimer with the androgen-responsive elements of target genes and their flanking DNA (Lobaccaro et al, 1996). The mechanism by which the receptor regulates gene transcription probably involves N-terminal sequences of the protein, but the molecular details of this activation process remain to be elucidated. Protein–protein interactions, probably with other transcription factors, may occur near the transcription start site of the gene. Both promoter and host cell specificity appear to influence the requirement for the N-terminal domain in transcriptional activation, suggesting that this region interacts with cell-specific transcription factors.

Male pseudohermaphroditism

Persistent Müllerian duct syndrome

Persistent Müllerian duct syndrome is usually discovered at surgery performed for cryptorchidism and/or hernia. It is a rare form of familial male pseudohermaphroditism, characterized by the persistence of the uterus and Fallopian tubes in 46,XY phenotypic males, and is due to defects in the synthesis or action of anti-Müllerian hormone (AMH) (Josso et al, 1993). Since the cloning and sequencing of both AMH and AMH-receptor genes, gene abnormalities have been described in patients with persistent Müllerian duct syndrome. Molecular genetics analyses have revealed a variety of mutations in the AMH gene covering the whole length of the gene (Imbeaud et al, 1994) but paradoxically affecting essentially the N-terminal region of the protein, which seems not to be essential to the bioactivity of the hormone.

Furthermore, one homozygous mutation of the AMH receptor has recently been described by Imbeaud et al (1995) in 1 AMH-positive patient out of 21 such patients. This splice mutation generated two abnormal mRNAs, one missing the second exon required for ligand binding, and the second coding for an abnormal protein due to an amino acid substitution followed by the insertion of four amino acids.

The treatment of persistent Müllerian duct syndrome is relatively straightforward in that all patients are phenotypic male and require orchidopexy.

Testosterone synthesis defect

Male pseudohermaphroditisms can be caused by a decrease in or an absence of androgen production due to an alteration of enzymes involved in the testosterone biosynthesis pathway (see Figure 1), whereas female pseudohermaphroditism results from an increased production of fetal androgens (Table 2).

Congenital lipoid adrenal hyperplasia. This is a rare disease characterized by a defect in the synthesis of the three classes of steroid hormone, resulting in severe salt wasting and a female phenotype. In humans, no mutation

Table 2. Clinical phenotype of testosterone biosynthesis abnormalities, protein involved and gene localization.

	Clinical form	Phenotype		Symptoms of aldosterone synthesis abnormality	Biological profile	Profile	Gene/location
		46,XX	46,XY				
Congenital lipoid hyperplasia		Female	Female	Salt-wasting	↓↓ Steroids	StAR	StAR/8p11.2
17α-Hydroxylase deficiency} 17-20-Desmolase deficiency}	Complete Partial	Female Female	Female AG	AHT AHT±	↑↑ P, DOC	P450c17	CYP17/10q24–25
3β-HSD deficiency	Complete Partial	AG AG	Female AG	Salt-wasting	↑↑ Δ5/Δ4 Steroids (basal and after stimulation)	3βHSDII	3βHSD-II/1p13
17β-HSD deficiency		Female	AG		↑↑ Δ4/T (basal and after stimulation)	17β-HSD-3	17β-HSD-3/9q22
21α-Hydroxylase deficiency	Salt-wasting Simple virilizing Non-classic	AG	Male	Salt-wasting	↑↑ 17-OHP (basal and/or after stimulation)	P450c21	CYP21B/6p21
11β-Hydroxylase deficiency		AG	Male	AHT	↑↑ 11-Deoxycortisol, DOC	P450c11B1	CYP11B1/8q22
Aromatase deficiency		AG	Male		↑↑ T/E2	P450arom	CYParo/15p21.1

has thus far been found in the gene encoding for P450scc, the first candidate gene, nor in the various proteins involved in cholesterol transport, such as SCP-2. Recently, the gene responsible for congenital lipoid adrenal hyperplasia has been cloned and validated by nonsense mutation (Lin et al, 1995). It encodes for a protein named StAR (steroidogenic acute regulatory protein), probably responsible for the transport of cholesterol to the inner membrane of mitochondria and thus to the P450scc enzyme complex.

17α-Hydroxylase deficiency. Defects in P450c17, which are frequently diagnosed at puberty, lead to a male pseudohermaphroditism with various degrees of ambiguous genitalia, most often a severe form associating female phenotype and hypertension. Cytochrome P450c17 catalyses the transformation of progesterone and pregnenolone into 17OH-progesterone and 17OH-pregnenolone (17α-hydroxylase activity) and then into dehydroepiandrosterone and Δ4-androstenedione (17-20-lyase activity).

The gene encoding for this enzymatic complex, the *CYP17* gene, is located on chromosome 10q24–25. Several different mutations have been reported in this gene, leading to either complete or partial forms of the disease (Yanase et al, 1991; Morel et al, 1995).

3β-Hydroxysteroid dehydrogenase deficiency. Defects in 3β-HSD functioning result in 46,XY individuals with male pseudohermaphroditism sometimes associated with salt-wasting in the classic form. The phenotype is variable and must be distinguished from the classic form of 21OH deficiency.

The 3β-HSD enzyme is responsible for the conversion of Δ5 (3βOH) steroids (pregnenolone, 17OH-pregnenolone, dehydroepiandrosterone, Δ5-androstenediol) into Δ4 (3-keto) steroids (progesterone, 17OH-progesterone, Δ4-androstenedione and testosterone respectively). Two different cDNAs have been identified: type I in placenta, and type II in gonads and adrenal glands. The two genes are located on chromosome 1p13. The two proteins are highly homologous and differ essentially by their tissue expression.

Almost 15 mutations of the type II 3β-HSD enzyme have been reported to date, but no mutation of type I has been found (Simard et al, 1993; Zhang et al, 1996). This can explain the virilization that occurs in 46,XX subjects, by a peripheral, non-steroidogenic conversion of elevated testosterone precursors.

A non-classic form of 3β-HSD deficiency has been described and is characterized by a late onset and less severe form of the disease. The clinical diagnosis of this form is not easy, and its existence remains controversial because no mutation of the gene has been found.

17β-Hydroxysteroid dehydrogenase deficiency. Type 3 17β-hydroxysteroid dehydrogenase deficiency is a rare autosomal recessive cause of male pseudohermaphroditism. The typical subject is a 46,XY male, born with female external genitalia and testes located in the inguinal canals or labia majora, who virilizes considerably at the time of puberty. The hormonal profile is characterized by elevated levels of androstenedione, contrasting with low or normal levels of testosterone. The deficiency in testosterone synthesis, associated with the well-differentiated Wolffian duct structures, is a puzzling characteristic of this disorder and may indicate that androgen must act by an alternative mechanism in these tissues in utero. As described for 5α-reductase deficiency, the pubertal virilization may result from extraglandular testosterone formation owing to a peripheral conversion of increased testicular androstenedione by unaffected 17β-HSD isoenzymes.

17β-hydroxysteroid dehydrogenase converts Δ4-androstenedione into testosterone, and dehydroepiandrosterone into androstenediol. It also acts on the interconversion of oestradiol and oestrone. This is a key enzyme leading to active androgenic compounds, and the only one in the steroido-genic pathway whose action is reversible. Three different enzymes with tissue-specific expression, encoded by three different genes, have been identified. The 17β-HSD type 1 has a peripheral activity and a specificity toward oestrogens. The 17β-HSD type 2 is mainly of placental origin and acts on both androgens and oestrogens. The 17β-HSD type 3 has a specific testicular expression and functions with NADPH as co-factor (unlike the two other enzymes, which utilize NADH). Finally, abnormalities of the type 3 enzyme are responsible for the 17β-HSD deficiency.

Among the gene alterations, missense and nonsense mutations, splice junction abnormalities and a small deletion that resulted in a frame shift have been described (Anderson et al, 1996). Expression of mutant enzymes after site-directed mutagenesis has shown that the missense mutations cause almost complete loss of enzymatic activity.

Affected newborns are considered to be female, but the sex of rearing remains open to question: the choice of sex will be influenced by the social group. We believe that when the female sex of rearing is maintained, orchidectomy must be carried out during infancy or childhood. If the diagnosis is not made prior to puberty, a gender change to male is acceptable.

Androgen resistance

5α-Reductase deficiency. Several investigators have reported a wide clinical, biological and biochemical spectrum associated with genetic heterogeneity in 5α-reductase deficiency. Diagnosis should be based on physical examination, pedigree analysis, analysis of basal and post-hCG stimulation plasma T and DHT levels, 5β/5α urinary steroid metabolite ratio, measurement of 5α-reductase activity in cultured genital skin fibro-blasts and finally analysis of the 5α-reductase 2 gene (Wilson et al, 1993).

Patients with 5α-reductase deficiency are characterized at birth by the presence of a pseudovagina, a urogenital sinus and testes in the inguinal canals, labia or scrotum in all cases (Table 3). The clinical presentation can range from almost normal female structures to a clear-cut male phenotype with hypospadias, bilateral testes and normal virilized Wolffian structures that terminate in the vagina. The main characteristic of 5α-reductase deficiency is the virilization of the external genitalia that occurs at puberty,

Table 3. Clinical phenotypes of androgen resistance.

		Androgen receptor disorders		
	5α-Reductase deficiency	Complete	Partial	Mild
External genitalia	Predominantly female	Female	Ambiguous	Male
Wolffian structures	Male	Absent	Hypoplastic male	Male
Urogenital sinus	Female	Female	Rudimentary male	Male
Breast	Male	Female	Gynaecomastia	±Gynaecomastia
Sexual orientation	Female→male	Female	Male/female	Male

along with the acquisition of male gender identity in these patients raised as female.

The characteristic endocrine features of 5α-reductase deficiency are normal-to-high levels of plasma testosterone and low levels of plasma dihydrotestosterone, elevation of the ratio of the concentration of plasma testosterone to dihydrotestosterone in adulthood and after stimulation with hCG in childhood, and elevated ratios of urinary 5β- to 5α metabolites of androgen and C21 steroids. The diagnosis of 5α-reductase deficiency is mainly supported by an increased T/DHT ratio.

From a biochemical point of view, the decrease in 5α-reductase activity in the intact genital skin fibroblasts supports the diagnosis of 5α-reductase deficiency, but enzymatic activity is sometimes within the normal range. The decreased activity in sonicated cell extracts at acidic pH provides strong evidence that the mutation results in a loss of type 2 enzyme activity.

Isolation and sequencing of the cDNA encoding the type 2 5α-reductase provides the molecular tools required for the definition of the gene abnormalities responsible for 5α-reductase deficiency. To date, only three gene deletions have been described (Wilson et al, 1993; Boudon et al, 1995a). Indeed, when a sequence alteration is identified, it is usually a point mutation. These mutations vary greatly and are found throughout the gene. To date, the standard methods of molecular genetic analysis have revealed two nonsense mutations, one splicing defect and 24 missense mutations (Jenkins et al, 1991; Wilson et al, 1993; Boudon et al, 1995b). Twelve of the missense mutations result in a protein with no detectable enzyme activity, whereas the remaining 10 give rise to proteins with severely decreased but measurable enzyme activity. The last group of mutations can be divided into two classes: those that affect the ability of the enzyme to bind testosterone substrate and those that decrease the affinity for the NADPH co-factor (Wigley et al, 1994).

The management of 5α-reductase deficiency is primarily dependent upon the phenotypic findings and gender at the time of diagnosis. Given the severe defect of the external genitalia, most newborns are raised as female. To prevent masculinization, gonadectomy should be performed early along with vaginoplasty and clitoral reduction. If the diagnosis is made in puberty, one can consider raising such a child as male: administration of supraphysiological doses of testosterone results in the long-term enhancement of virilization.

Androgen insensitivity syndrome. Initially described by Morris in 1953, androgen insensitivity syndromes have been divided into two groups from a clinical point of view—complete and partial androgen insensitivity (Table 3).

Complete androgen insensitivity is characterized by an unambiguous female phenotype with a blind vaginal pouch and no uterus. In some cases, an underdevelopment of the clitoris and labia minora may be observed. At puberty, breast development is normal or augmented, contrasting with the absent or scanty axillary and pubic hair in the majority of cases. Moreover, patients with complete androgen insensitivity develop a female habitus. Individuals with complete androgen insensitivity come to medical attention during infancy because of the development of inguinal hernia, or during puberty because of a primary amenorrhoea.

Partial androgen insensitivity covers a wide spectrum of clinical phenotypes from patients with an essentially female phenotype, with limited evidence of androgenization, such as mild clitoromegaly and/or a small degree of posterior labial fusion, to infertile individuals who had normal responsiveness during fetal life and thus an unequivocally male phenotype with azoospermia. Diagnosis is made in infancy from ambiguous genitalia, 46,XY karyotype and endocrine features. At puberty, virilization and/or feminization may occur depending on the hormonal profile of the patient.

Since the androgen receptor gene has been cloned, the tools of molecular biology have made it possible to identify mutations within the androgen receptor gene from patients with different phenotypes of androgen insensitivity (see Figure 3) (Quigley et al, 1995). Such techniques include restriction fragment length polymorphism analysis and enzymatic amplification of the various exons of the androgen receptor gene to detect large-scale changes in the gene structure. Screening procedures with sequencing of the gene allow the identification of subtle changes responsible for missense or nonsense mutations. Measurements of androgen receptor mRNA have been useful in identifying mutations that cause androgen insensitivity by altering the levels or the size of the mRNA. Transfection of constructs expressing the mutant androgen receptor in mammalian cells is the main approach for demonstrating the causative role of the mutation in the development of the androgen insensitivity.

Androgen receptor gene alterations may be classified into two groups according to the DNA and mRNA alterations: (a) loss or gain of genomic information, such as macro and microdeletions and base pair insertions, and (b) point mutations, responsible for nonsense, missense and splice mutations. Molecular genetic analysis of the androgen receptor gene has revealed that there is a wide variety of molecular defects underlying the clinical and biochemical heterogeneity of androgen insensitivity syndrome. All androgen receptor defects appear to disturb the ability of the androgen receptor to regulate transcription of its target genes, although androgen receptor gene sequencing and in vitro studies of receptor function do not explain every aspect of androgen insensitivity. Moreover, the same mutation can be associated with different phenotypes even within the same family. Markedly different molecular defects (major deletion, premature termination, single amino acid substitution in the protein) can produce the same phenotype. It thus seems that other genetic determinants may influence the action of androgen within its target cells.

The screening of carriers and the prenatal diagnosis of androgen insensitivity in high-risk families is impossible unless the mutation has been identified (Figure 5). Once the mutation has been described and correlated to the disease, sequencing of the suspected exon of the 46,XX siblings or the 46,XY fetus determines whether they are carrying an affected chromosome (Lumbroso et al, 1994). However, when the mutation has not been identified, it is necessary to look for one of the two androgen receptor gene polymorphisms (Lobaccaro et al, 1992, 1994).

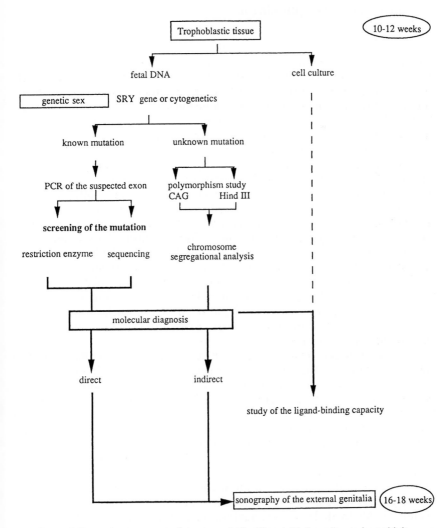

Figure 5. Prenatal management of pregnancy in families at risk for androgen insensitivity.

The treatment of patients with complete androgen insensitivity syndrome relates primarily to the optional timing of gonadectomy. We perform gonadectomy before puberty and prescribe oestrogens during puberty. The management of patients with partial androgen insensitivity syndrome must be individualized depending on the degree of genital ambiguity, the growth response of the penis to supraphysiological doses of testosterone and the type of androgen receptor mutation. Although certain androgen receptor defects may be amenable to androgen therapy, multiple interventions for the reconstruction of external genitalia and azoospermia are good arguments for a female sex of rearing.

Female pseudohermaphroditism

Testosterone synthesis excess

21α-Hydroxylase deficiency. (see also Chapter 4). In classic 21-hydroxylase deficiency, high plasma concentrations of androgens, due to precursor diversion, cause virilization of the external genitalia of the 46,XX female fetus early in gestation. This deficiency is the most common cause of female pseudohermaphroditism. About 75% of patients with classic 21-hydroxylase deficiency do not correctly synthesize aldosterone, which induces a potentially fatal salt-wasting (New, 1995).

In this congenital adrenal hyperplasia, 17α-hydroxyprogesterone is not converted effectively to 11-deoxycortisol in the pathway of cortisol synthesis. Owing to the enzymatic defect, the aldosterone pathway is also impaired because of the absence or reduced conversion of progesterone to 11-deoxycorticosterone. The classic form (salt-wasting and simple virilizing) has a frequency estimated at 1 in 14 000 live births. The definitive test to diagnose classic 21-hydroxylase deficiency is a standard ACTH stimulation test and measurement of plasma 17α-hydroxyprogesterone. A variant of 21-hydroxylase deficiency, due to a milder enzymatic effect, is the non-classic form of the disease. Affected females do not present neonatal genital ambiguity but rather other signs of androgen excess, such as hirsutism. In contrast to the classic form, non-classic 21-hydroxylase deficiency occurs at a frequency of 1 in 100.

The *CYP21B* gene encoding 21-hydroxylase is located on the short arm of chromosome 6 in the HLA complex (Figure 6). *CYP21B* and its pseudogene *CYP21A* alternate with two genes, *C4A* and *C4B*, encoding the fourth component of serum complement. Because the two *CYP21* genes, which contain 10 exons each, are approximately 98% identical, gene deletion and apparent gene conversion are frequent events, causing 21-hydroxylase deficiency. *CYP21B* gene deletions account for 10–35% of abnormal alleles (Ghanem et al, 1990; White and New, 1992). The majority of the point mutations described in the *CYP21B* gene result from microgene conversion, i.e. short sequences on the pseudogene that are transferred to the active gene (Figure 6). The mechanism of gene conversion is still not completely understood. However, analysis in matched sperm and peripheral blood leukocyte DNA samples from normal individuals has suggested that

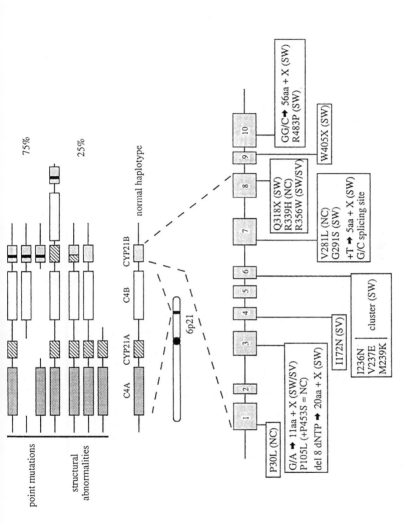

Figure 6. Schematic representation of the *CYP/C4* cluster gene organization. Structural abnormalities and point mutations described in 21-hydroxylase deficiency. Adapted from White and New (1992) and completed with mutations described more recently. NC, non-classic form; SW, salt wasting form; SV, simple-virilizing form.

whereas deletions occur exclusively in meiosis, gene conversions occur during both meiosis and mitosis, or perhaps only during mitosis (Tusie-Luna and White, 1995). Thus gene conversions must occur by a mechanism distinct from unequal crossing-over. Although, a genotype–phenotype relationship has been noted, it seems that the genotype does not always predict the phenotype, even within the same family.

Prenatal diagnosis is important to identify the enzymatic defiency so that genital ambiguity in affected females can be prevented by proper dexamethasone treatment of the pregnant mother (Speiser and New, 1994). This prenatal diagnosis can be hormonal, by the measurement of amniotic fluid 17α-progesterone levels, or genetic, after chorionic villus sampling at 9–10 weeks of gestation. Proper prenatal diagnosis and treatment of 21-hydroxylase deficiency thus spares the newborn female the consequences of genital ambiguity, sex misassignment and gender confusion (Figure 7).

11β-Hydroxylase deficiency. Female newborns usually present with signs of androgen excess, such as masculinization of the external genitalia. Many

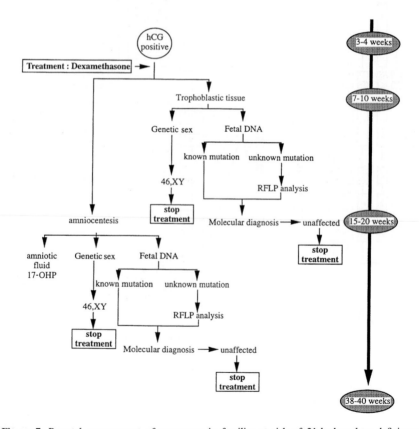

Figure 7. Prenatal management of pregnancy in families at risk of 21-hydroxylase deficiency. Adapted from New (1995).

patients also develop signs and symptoms of aldosterone deficiency, including hyponatraemia, hyperkalaemia and hypovolaemia, which induce salt-wasting. Only a small percentage of patients develop hypertension rather than mineralocorticoid deficiency.

This enzymatic deficiency, which fails to convert 11-deoxycortisol to cortisol, is the second most common cause of congenital adrenal hyperplasia and results in a hypertensive form of the disease. Humans have two isoenzymes with 11β-hydroxylase activity that are required for cortisol and aldosterone synthesis. CYP11B1, which carries the 11β-hydroxylase activity, is regulated by ACTH, and CYP11B2, which carries the aldosterone synthetase activity, is regulated by angiotensin II. Moreover, in addition to the 11β-hydroxylase activity, the latter enzyme has 18-hydroxylase and 18-oxidase activities and can thus synthesize aldosterone from deoxycorticosterone.

Deficiency of 11β-hydroxylase results from mutations in the *CYP11B1* gene. All mutations identified in patients with the classic form abolish enzymatic activity (White et al, 1994). However, there is no consistent correlation between the severity of hypertension and the degree of virilization in individuals with the same homozygous mutation. These phenotypic variations may be due to factors outside the *CYP11B1* gene locus.

The treatment of affected children with hydrocortisone achieves a number of goals, while feminizing genitoplasty must be performed at 6–12 months of age.

3β-Hydroxysteroid deshydrogenase deficiency. The complete form of 3β-hydroxysteroid deshydrogenase deficiency results in partially virilized external genitalia in genetic females, whereas a partial form results in adolescent hyperandrogenism. Salt-losing is present when the deficiency is complete. An elevated secretion of pregnenolone and 17α-pregnenolone is characteristic of this form of congenital adrenal hyperplasia (Simard et al, 1993; Zhang et al, 1996).

Hydrocortisone and salt-retaining hormone replacement therapy are needed.

Oestrogen synthesis defect: aromatase deficiency

Aromatase deficiency within placental syncytiotrophoblasts is responsible for impaired or absent conversion of fetal and maternal androgens to oestrogens. It subsequently leads, in the mother, to the development of signs of hyperandrogenism (acne and hirsutism) during the second half of pregnancy. Exposure of the female fetus to this androgen excess causes virilization of the infant, with severe ambiguous genitalia—micropenis, hypospadias, and posterior labioscrotal fusion—at birth. At puberty, affected females present with pubertal failure, hypergonadotropic hypogonadism, virilization and histological and biological signs similar to those observed in polycystic ovarian syndrome, but in aromatase deficiency, oestrogen levels are exceedingly low. In both sexes, it leads to delayed bone age and tall stature.

Several mutations within the *P450arom* gene have been described in the past few years (Morishima et al, 1995). The descriptions of aromatase deficiency in male and female provide new insights into the physiological role of oestrogens during pregnancy, puberty, the bone maturation and turnover process, and the sex steroid-gonadotropin feedback mechanism in the male.

SUMMARY

In conclusion, the cloning of the genes responsible for sexual determination and sexual differentiation has proved useful for analysing ambiguous genitalia and for clarifying the genetic defect underlying male and female pseudohermaphroditisms. Moreover, molecular genetics analysis can also be used for carrier identification and prenatal diagnosis. Molecular analysis of ambiguous genitalia is a good model for obtaining further knowledge on human sex determination and sexual differentiation.

REFERENCES

Andersson S, Geissler WM, Wu L et al (1996) Molecular genetics and pathophysiology of 17β-hydroxysteroid dehydrogenase 3 deficiency. *Journal of Clinical Endocrinology and Metabolism* **81:** 130–136.

Bardoni B, Zanaria E, Guioli G et al (1994) A dosage sensitive locus at chromosome Xp21 is involved in male to male sex reversal. *Nature Genetics* **7:** 497–501.

Berta P, Hawkins JR, Sinclair AH et al (1990) Genetic evidence equating SRY and the testis-determining factor. *Nature* **348:** 448–450.

Boudon C, Lobaccaro J, Lumbroso S et al (1995a) A new deletion of the 5α-reductase type 2 gene in a Turkish family with 5α-reductase deficiency. *Clinical Endocrinology* **43:** 183–188.

Boudon C, Lumbroso S, Lobaccaro JM et al (1995b) Molecular study of the 5 alpha-reductase type 2 gene in three European families with 5 alpha-reductase deficiency. *Journal of Clinical Endocrinology and Metabolism* **80:** 2149–2153.

Brinkmann AO (1994) Steroid hormone receptors: activators of gene transcription. *Journal of Pediatric Endocrinology* **7:** 275–282.

Ghanem N, Lobaccaro J-M, Burési C et al (1990) Defective, deleted or converted CYP21B gene and negative association with a rare restriction fragment length polymorphism allele of the factor B gene in congenital adrenal hyperplasia. *Human Genetics* **86:** 117–125.

Imbeaud S, Rey R, Carré-Eusèbe D et al (1994) Molecular genetics of the persistent Müllerian duct syndrome: a study of 19 families. *Human Molecular Genetics* **3:** 125–131.

Imbeaud S, Faure E, Lamarre I et al (1995) Insensitivity to anti-Müllerian hormone due to a mutation in the human anti-Müllerian hormone receptor. *Nature Genetics* **11:** 382–388.

Hawkins JR (1993) The SRY gene. *Trends in Endocrinology and Metabolism* **4:** 328–332.

Jenkins EP, Andersson S, Imperato McGinley J et al (1991) Genetic and pharmacological evidence for more than one human steroid 5α-reductase. *Journal of Clinical Investigation* **89:** 293–300.

Josso N, Cate RL & Picard JY (1993) Anti-Müllerian factor: the Jost factor. In Bardin CW (ed.) *Recent Progress in Hormone Research*, pp 1–59. San Diego: Academic Press.

Koopman P, Gubbay J, Vivian N et al (1991) Male development of chromosomally female mice transgenic for SRY. *Nature* **351:** 117–121.

Kremer H, Kraaij R, Toledo SPA et al (1995) Male pseudohermaphroditism due to a homozygous missense mutation of the luteinizing hormone receptor gene. *Nature Genetics* **9:** 160–164.

Lin D, Sugawara T, Staruss JF III et al (1995) Role of steroidogenic acute regulatory protein in adrenal and gonadal steroidogenesis. *Science* **267:** 1828–1831.

Lobaccaro JM, Lumbroso S, Carré-Pigeon F et al (1992) Prenatal prediction of androgen insensitivity syndrome using exon 1 polymorphism of the androgen receptor gene. *Journal of Steroid Biochemistry and Molecular Biology* **43:** 659–663.

Lobaccaro J-M, Belon C, Lumbroso S et al (1994) Molecular prenatal diagnosis of partial androgen insensitivity syndrome based on the Hind III polymorphism of the androgen receptor gene. *Clinical Endocrinology* **40:** 297–302.

Lobaccaro JM, Poujol N, Chiche L et al (1996) Molecular modeling and *in vitro* investigations of the human androgen receptor DNA-binding domain: application for the study of two mutations. *Molecular and Cellular Endocrinology* **116:** 137–147.

Lumbroso S, Lobaccaro JM, Belon C et al (1994) Molecular prenatal exclusion of Reifenstein syndrome. *European Journal of Endocrinology* **130:** 327–332.

Morel Y, Mebarki F & Portrat S (1995) Génétique des pseudohermaphrodismes masculins par anomalies de la synthèse de la testostérone. In Chaussain JL & Roger M (eds) *Les ambiguïtés sexuelles*, pp 53–75. Paris: SEPE.

Morishima A, Grumbach MM, Simpson ER et al (1995) Aromatase deficiency in male and female siblings caused by a novel mutation and the physiological role of estrogens. *Journal of Clinical Endocrinology and Metabolism* **80:** 3689–3698.

Morris JM (1953) The syndrome of testicular feminization in male pseudohermaphrodites. *American Journal of Obstetrics and Gynecology* **65:** 1192–1211.

Muscatelli F, Strom TM, Walker AP et al (1994) Mutations in the DAX-1 gene give rise to both X-linked adrenal hypoplasia congenita and hypogonadotropic hypogonadism. *Nature.* **372:** 672–676.

New MI (1995) Steroid 21-hydroxylase deficiency (congenital adrenal hyperplasia). *American Journal of Medicine* **98(S1A):** 2S–8S.

Palmer MS, Sinclair AH, Berta P et al (1989) Genetic evidence that ZFY is not the testis-determining factor. *Nature* **342:** 937–939.

Quigley CA, Debellis A, Marschke KB et al (1995) Androgen receptor defects: historical, clinical, and molecular perspectives. *Endocrine Reviews* **16:** 271–321.

Simard J, Rheaume E, Sanchez R et al (1993) Molecular basis of congenital adrenal hyperplasia due to 3β-hydroxysteroid dehydrogenase defiency. *Molecular Endocrinology* **7:** 716–728.

Sinclair AH, Berta P, Palmer MS et al (1990) A gene from the human sex-determining region encodes a protein with homology to a conserved DNA-binding motif. *Nature* **346:** 240–244.

Speiser PW & New MI (1994) Prenatal diagnosis and treatment of congenital adrenal hyperplasia. *Journal of Pediatric Endocrinology* **7:** 183–191.

Sultan C, Lobaccaro JM, Lumbroso S et al (1995) Molecular aspects of sex differentiation—applications in pathological conditions. In Bergada C & Moguilevsky JA (eds) *Frontiers in Endocrinology. Puberty: Basic and Clinical Aspects*, pp 21–35. Roma: Serono Symposia Publications.

Tusie-Luna MT & White PC (1995) Gene conversions and unequal crossovers between CYP21 (steroid 21-hydroxylase gene) and CYP21P involve different mechanisms. *Proceedings of the National Academy of Science of the USA* **92:** 10 796–10 800.

Wagner T, Wirth J, Meyer J et al (1994) Autosomal sex reversal and campomelic dysplasia are caused by mutations in and around the SRY-related gene SOX9. *Cell* **79:** 1111–1120.

White PC & New MI (1992) Genetic basis of endocrine disease 2: congenital adrenal hyperplasia due to 21-hydroxylase deficiency. *Journal of Clinical Endocrinology and Metabolism* **74:** 6–11.

White PC, Curnow KM & Pascoe L (1994) Disorders of steroid 11β-hydroxylase isozymes. *Endocrinology Review* **15:** 421–438.

Wigley WC, Prihoda JS, Mowszowicz I et al (1994) Natural mutagenesis study of the human steroid 5 alpha-reductase 2 isozyme. Biochemistry. **33:** 1265–1270.

Wilson JD, Griffin JE & Russell DW (1993) Steroid 5α-reductase 2 deficiency. *Endocrinology Review* **14:** 577–593.

Yanase T, Simpson ER & Waterman MR (1991) 17alpha-hydroxylase/17,20-lyase deficiency—from clinical investigation to molecular definition. *Endocrine Review* **12:** 91–108.

Zhang L, Sakkal-Alkaddour H, Chang YT et al (1996) A new compound heterozygous frameshift mutation in the type II 3β-hydroxysteroid dehydrogenase (3β-HSD) gene causes salt-wasting 3β-HSD deficency congenital adrenal hyperplasia. *Journal of Clinical Endocrinology and Metabolism* **81:** 291–295.

2

Pathophysiology and consequences of intrauterine growth retardation

PAUL CZERNICHOW

Intrauterine growth retardation (IUGR) is the consequence of fetal mal-nutrition. IUGR infants have a higher than average risk of morbidity and mortality. Although most infants show some degree of catch-up growth during the first years of life, they may show persistent short stature later in life. Long-term consequences of IUGR, such as hypertension, diabetes and increased risk of cardiovascular and cerebrovascular disease, have also been described in adults (Barker et al, 1993). This emphasizes the import-ance of a clear understanding of the mechanisms regulating growth in normal human fetuses and in conditions such as intrauterine malnutrition.

HORMONAL REGULATION OF NORMAL AND PATHOLOGICAL FETAL GROWTH

At the start of gestation, growth appears to be controlled by nutritional input and growth factors acting locally by autocrine or paracrine mechanisms.

Among these, the insulin-like growth factors (IGFs) and their binding proteins (IGFBPs), modulating their action at the cellular level, play an important role during the different cellular phases of embryogenesis: mitosis, differentiation, selective recognition of cells among themselves, migration and programmed cell death or apoptosis (for a review, see Jones and Clemmons, 1995). Transgenetic experiments in the mouse reveal that the absence of expression of the gene for IGF-II is associated at birth with an anomaly in fetoplacental development without the presence of morpho-logical abnormalities (DeChiara et al, 1990). The absence of expression of the gene for IGF-I and/or its receptor leads to an anomaly in fetal growth and elevated neonatal mortality associated, according to the authors, with problems of differentiation most predominant at the muscular and gonadal levels (Baker et al, 1993; Liu et al, 1993). Thus, IGF-II seems to play an essential mitogenic role precociously in organogenesis, and IGF-I possibly a later role, with effects on cellular differentiation and growth.

Later on, once fetal circulation has become established, three separate compartments can be distinguished: maternal, placental and fetal. Each one

Baillière's Clinical Paediatrics—
Vol. 4, No. 2, May 1996
ISBN 0–7020–2180–6
0963–6714/96/020245 + 13 $12.00/00

of these compartments plays a major role. They elaborate distinct growth factors and play differing roles in energy transfers, thus influencing fetal growth.

Maternal factors

In the final stage of gestation, fetal growth is limited by maternal phenotype, in the size and quality of the uterine environment. This major point is well illustrated by the reduction in birthweight and length of babies of multiple pregnancies.

During pregnancy, the maternal hormonal profile is greatly changed by the influence of placental hormones such as human chorionic gonadotrophin (hCG), human placental lactogen (hPL) and placental growth hormone (which will be discussed later) being liberated into the maternal compartment. The principal somatotrophic factors, IGF-I, IGF-II and maternal insulin, do not cross the placental barrier and therefore play no direct role on fetal growth. They do, however, play an important role in the modification of placental function, thus influencing the distribution of nutrients between the fetus and the placenta. In the mouse, the administration of IGF-I to the mother increases fetal growth and modifies the ratio of fetal to placental growth, to the disadvantage of the latter (Gluckman et al, 1992a). The maternal IGF-I levels increase throughout pregnancy and can be correlated with fetal growth (Mirlesse et al, 1993).

Placental factors

The placenta has a number of functions essential for the survival and development of the fetus. Nutrients, oxygen, water and macromolecules that are indispensible for fetoplacental development are transferred by an exchange process between the microvillar surface of the syncytiotrophoblast and the maternal blood system. The syncytiotrophoblast is, furthermore, a unique endocrine organ secreting steroids, peptide hormones such as hCG, hCS (human chorionic somatomammotrophin), sometimes called hPL (human placental lactogen), placental growth hormone (placental GH), growth factors and cytokines, which are implicated by paracrine or autocrine mechanisms in fetoplacental growth (Évain-Brion, 1992).

Despite the key role of the placenta in fetal growth, little is yet known about the regulation of its implantation and growth or the development of placental functions. Recent data show a role for IGF-I and its binding protein IGFBP-1 in the implantation process (Giudice et al, 1994), and for ligands of the epidermal growth factor (EGF) receptor in syncytial differentiation (Alsat et al, 1993). The EGF receptor is impaired in the placentae of intrauterine growth-retarded cases (Fondacci et al, 1994; Gabriel et al, 1994).

It has been known for a number of years that the placenta liberates very high levels of hPL (hCS) into the maternal compartment and 100 times less into the fetal circulation. However, besides a possible metabolic role for the maintenance of glucose input to the fetus in case of prolonged fasting, there is no direct clinical evidence of a role for this hormone in fetal growth. Numerous examples have been described of normal fetal growth in spite of deletion of the hPL gene. On the other hand, recent studies underline the importance of the role played by placental growth hormone, specifically expressed in the syncytiotrophoblast (Frankenne et al, 1990; Scippo et al, 1992). This hormone progressively replaces maternal hypophyseal growth hormone, which falls to undetectable levels during the second trimester of pregnancy (Frankenne et al, 1988; Mirlesse et al, 1993). Secreted at constant levels by the placenta, it seems to regulate maternal IGF-I levels. The latter are effectively correlated with placental GH levels. Furthermore, in pathology, maternal IGF-I increases progressively during the pregnancies of acromegalic women, thus following the level of placental GH, depite high stable levels of hypophyseal GH (Beckers et al, 1990). Finally, the levels of placental GH and IGF-I are lowered in women carrying a fetus showing IUGR (Mirlesse et al, 1993). The secretion of placental GH, but not that of hPL or hCG, is inhibited in vitro by glucose in explants of trophoblastic cells (Patel et al, 1995). This suggests a metabolic role for placental GH specifically secreted into the maternal compartment and undetected in fetal circulation. In the case of lowered maternal glycaemia, the placental GH then abundantly secreted by the placenta would maintain the energy input to the fetus (Frankenne et al, 1992). A further direct role for placental GH on the development of the placenta, as well as on its multiple endocrine and immunological functions, cannot be excluded.

Fetal factors

GH is found at high levels in fetal circulation; its secretion is regulated by the neuroendocrine mechanisms described in the adult. The exact reasons for the elevated fetal plasma concentration are unclear—predominance of positive hypothalamic stimulation is one possible explanation. An alternative explanation is the lack of inhibitory feedback by the low concentration of circulating IGF-I. As shown by De Zegher (De Zegher et al, 1988), IGF-I administration to the ovine fetus, which has low IGF-I concentrations during fetal life, results in a sharp decline in plasma GH values in the fetal compartment, a result in favour of this hypothesis.

Furthermore, GH receptors are present in fetal tissue at the end of gestation (Hill et al, 1992). It has generally been considered that GH plays little if any role in fetal growth because fetal pituitary ablation or anencephaly are reported to have little effect on fetal size (Gluckman et al, 1981). However, recent studies of neonates with congenital GH deficiency have clearly shown that these infants have reduced birth length and progressive growth failure in early postnatal life (Gluckman et al, 1992b). Therefore GH plays a role in perinatal and infantile growth, although it is not the key hormone for fetal growth.

On the other hand, insulin is certainly a major element in the control of fetal growth, which is severely impaired by pancreatic agenesis (Lemons et al, 1979). Furthermore, the secondary hyperinsulinism seen in the fetuses of diabetic mothers is accompanied by predominant hypertrophy of the adipose tissue mass, reflecting the direct lipogenic effects of insulin. However, it is always difficult to differentiate in the role of insulin its direct somatotrophic effects from the indirect effects related to the metabolic changes it induces. Thus, in the sheep, an increase in fetal insulinaemia with no parallel increase of substrate input has no effect on fetal growth (Fowden et al, 1989). It is also possible that insulin stimulates fetal growth by increasing the production of IGF-I.

Recent studies effectively suggest a particular role for the IGFs in fetal growth. A direct role for IGF-I has been clearly shown in the mouse by transgenetic experiments previously cited and embryo transfer. Fetuses showing constitutively high IGF-I levels grow faster than do those showing lower levels (Kroonsberg et al, 1989). In human pathology, fetuses showing IUGR have low levels of IGF-I associated with modifications in the profile of binding proteins (Leger et al, 1996a,b) (Table 1). This growth factor, which in postnatal life is regulated by GH, seems to be modulated during fetal life mainly by nutritional status, particularly the glucose input to the fetus. Thus, in the sheep, maternal fasting leads to a drop in fetal IGF-I levels that can be normalized by an infusion of glucose or insulin, but not of amino acids (Oliver et al, 1993). In the same way, in this animal model, IGF-I injection increases fetal captation of glucose and protein synthesis, and inhibits the production of placental lactate. Fetal IGF-I therefore seems to distribute energy input between the placenta and the fetus for the greater benefit of the fetus. However, in the fetus showing IUGR, the concentration of the binding protein IGFBP-3 is low towards the end of gestation and in cord blood. This, associated with the low concentrations of IGF-I, characterizes a state of resistance to GH, as shown by elevated

Table 1. Plasma concentrations of IGF-I, IGFBP-3 and GH in a population of fetuses at different stages of gestation and in newborn infants whose intrauterine development was marked by a growth retardation (IUGR), in comparison with subjects showing normal development (control). Adapted from Leger et al (1996a,b).

		18–29 weeks	30–40 weeks	Cord blood	1 month
IGF-I	IUGR	31.6 +/– 2.9	49.1 +/– 3.8	32.0 +/– 21.0	79.0 +/– 33.0
(ng/ml) +/– SD		***	***	****	
		$n = 36$	$n = 24$	$n = 14$	$n = 125$
	Control	41.5 +/– 1.7	66.4 +/– 31.0	85.0 +/– 38.0	90.0 +/– 35.0
		$n = 92$	$n = 71$	$n = 44$	$n = 51$
IGFBP-3	IUGR	1.28 +/– 0.1	1.36 +/– 0.5	1.2 +/– 0.9	1.8 +/– 0.5
(ng/ml) +/– SD			**	*	
		$n = 31$	$n = 24$	$n = 44$	$n = 125$
	Control	1.39 +/– 0.08	1.69 +/– 0.18	1.5 +/– 0.4	1.7 +/– 0.7
		$n = 83$	$n = 66$	$n = 44$	$n = 51$
GH	IUGR	41 +/– 5.1	23.4 +/– 3.1	46.0 +/– 44.0	12.0 +/– 8.0
(ng/ml) +/– SD		$n = 30$	$n = 21$	$n = 173$	$n = 125$
	Control	33.6 +/– 2.1	21.9 +/– 1.4	19.9	10.0 +/– 8.0
		$n = 82$	$n = 65$	$n = 44$	$n = 51$

$* P = 0.02; ** P = 0.05; *** P = 0.02; **** P = 0.001.$

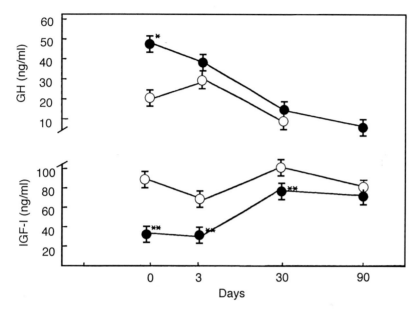

Figure 1. Evolution of plasma concentrations of IGF-I and GH during the first months of postnatal life in a group of infants with IUGR (●) and in a control group (○). GH levels are elevated, whereas IGF-I levels are very low in the cord blood of infants having suffered from intrauterine malnutrition. These parameters are rapidly corrected during the first weeks of postnatal life. * $P < 0.0005$; ** $P < 0.0001$. Adapted from Leger et al (1996a).

plasma GH concentrations (Leger et al, 1966a,b; Lassare et al, 1991). Since a feedback mechanism is operational at the end of gestation between GH and IGF-I, it is equally possible that low levels of IGF-I are also responsible for high GH concentrations in the fetal compartment. As soon as the child is removed from the intrauterine conditions responsible for malnutrition, and renutrition is achieved in appropriate conditions, a rapid increase of IGF-I and a decrease in GH (Leger et al, 1996a) levels is observed. At the end of the first trimester of life, the infant shows normal secretion of growth factors and GH (Figure 1; Table 1 above).

Conclusion

Harmonious fetal growth depends on a perfect balance between the different development factors from the maternal, fetal and placental compartments. The key role of the latter in fetal growth should be stressed. Any pathology interfering with trophoblastic invasion, and/or syncytial differentiation, will have major repercussions on fetal growth, such as have been observed in the case of toxaemia of pregnancy or pre-eclampsia.

Whatever the cause, growth retardation is due in the majority of cases to a major default in nutritional input to the fetus. The lowering of growth factor levels, particularly that of fetal IGF-I, is a consequence of this intrauterine malnutrition. Whether the growth retardation will be reversible during postnatal life is difficult to predict. A better knowledge of the different factors that control the reversibility is absolutely necessary for the establishment of a rational attitude in the surveillance of these pregnancies. For the time being, we have to rely on difficult estimations that provide only an approximate guide to the obstetrician in taking a decision in favour of a premature delivery to remove the fetus from an unfavourable intra-uterine environment.

CLINICAL ASPECTS OF IUGR

Definition and causes

IUGR is defined as that giving rise to a weight or length inferior to the reference normal values for a given gestation age.

As a general rule, authors choose the 10th or the 3rd percentile, or the 2nd standard deviation of the reference curves with respect to the normal values, to define IUGR. This variability in the definition of the condition naturally introduces a certain difficulty into the comparative analysis of different studies. Most of the published work uses weight as the criterion for IUGR.

The association of late development in both weight and length defines a symmetrical or harmonious growth retardation. This is the result of pro-longed and more severe intrauterine malnutrition, and gives rise to a more pessimistic prognosis. In a study of 258 infants showing IUGR with a birthweight inferior to the 3rd percentile, 63% also showed severe retardation with respect to length (Thizon de Gaulle, 1992). In a study of 3650 newborn infants, Karlberg and Albertsson-Wikland (1995) found 5.4% of them to have a weight and/or length inferior to the 2nd standard deviation. In this study, 1.6% and 2.4% showed respectively a weight or a length inferior to this limit, and 1.5% associated the two parameters (symmetrical growth retardation). Those newborn infants with symmetrical growth retardation affecting both length and weight seem to have a less favourable prognosis than those showing an asymmetrical growth retardation affecting only weight. In fact, two elements seem to be important in the ultimate prognosis: the severity of damage to the cranial circumference, which can only slightly be caught up after growth, and the importance of the statural delay, which conditions the height after 2 years of age (see below).

Intrauterine malnutrition not only affects the growth in length or in weight of the newborn infant, but also interferes with the normal develop-ment of various organs. Naeye et al (1973) have studied organ weights of a large cohort of stillborn and liveborn infants who died from various causes. Maternal undernutrition had a profound effect not only on body size, but also on organ growth: liver, adrenal glands, kidneys and placenta were very notably affected.

The growth of the kidney has been particularly studied. We know, for example, that in the human, severe IUGR is accompanied by a decrease in size of the kidneys, both in a group of third trimester stillbirths and in infants who died during the first year of life (Honchcliffe et al, 1992). More importantly, in the latter postnatal group, the number of glomeruli was decreased: there were only 65% of the number of glomeruli measured in a control group. Similar observations have been made in animal models (Merlet-Benichou et al, 1993). The effect of fetal malnutrition on the individual growth of each organ is still poorly understood and is probably of major importance in the postnatal morbidity of these infants. A systematic review of other organs, such as the lung, heart and adrenal glands, which develop in a rapid fashion during late gestation, is needed. Such findings would provide support for the point of view of certain obstetricians that prenatal therapy or elective pre-term delivery of affected fetuses should be considered to facilitate resumption of development by the improvement of general fetal conditions.

The principal known causes of IUGR are maternal elevated blood pressure (particularly in its most dangerous form, that of toxaemia of pregnancy), placental abnormalities, nutritional problems and maternal intoxication (alcohol, tobacco and drugs). In France, at least 25% of IUGR cases are due to maternal arterial hypertension and tobacco, the two factors often being associated (Thizon de Gaulle et al, 1992). The major role played by elevated blood pressure in the genesis of IUGR must be emphasized, as preventive measures are possible. It has been shown that aspirin, in low doses, has a preventive effect on growth retardation in the fetus (Uzan et al, 1991).

CONSEQUENCES OF IUGR

This review cannot undertake a detailed analysis of the acute metabolic consequences and the long-term neurosensorial results of fetal malnutrition. We must recall that the perinatal mortality statistics in these cases are five times greater than those of control newborn infants of identical gestational age (Koops, 1978). These results, already outdated, have been improved by decisions to remove fetuses in situations of distress, by better neonatal care, by prevention and treatment of acidosis, hypoglycaemia and hypocalcaemia, and, in a general manner, by better nutritional surveillance.

The consequences of new obstetric strategies on long-term neurosensory sequelae should also be evaluated. We can say, in general terms, that the neuromotor and sensory prognoses are closely related to cranial circumference, hence the importance of close surveillance of this parameter in a fetus suffering from growth retardation (Koops, 1978; Ounsted et al, 1989).

Postnatal growth

The postnatal growth of infants born with IUGR is characterized by a rate of growth designated as catch-up, i.e. a rate of growth superior to that seen in the normal infant. This phenomenon intervenes precociously, in the first months of life, and is more or less prolonged. This 'catch-up' affects first the weight then the length, and means that at the end of the second year, a normal size has in the majority of cases been attained.

We can see in Figure 2 the evolution of the weight, height and head circumference in a group of infants studied longitudinally for 2 years. Those infants having a birth length below −2 standard deviations have at the age of 2 a height situated within normal limits. This study illustrates the catch-up possibilities of these infants who, thanks to a growth rate superior to the norm, will have made up nearly 2 standard deviations within 2 years.

However, a certain number of children will remain small. According to published studies, 10–35% of the infants have at the age of 2–5 years a major statural handicap, with a height inferior to the 2nd standard deviation below average (Fitzhardinge and Steven, 1972; Francourt et al, 1976; Davies, 1981; Ounsted et al, 1982; Tenovuo et al, 1987; Fitzhardinge and Inwood, 1989). These studies indicate that prematurity and a pronounced degree of statural deficiency at birth are elements of poor prognosis. It seems surprising that there is so much variation between studies in the evaluation of the statural possibilites of infants born with IUGR. In fact, the series are often ill-matched, concerning children from homes of very different socio-economic status and those whose postnatal follow-up is

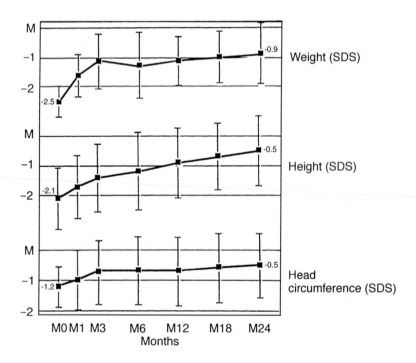

Figure 2. Evolution of the weight, height and occipitofrontal head circumference in a population of children born with IUGR. At 2 years, the average weight and height fall within the normal zone. The head circumference does not progress as favourably. M = mean; SDS = standard deviation score. Adapted from Thizon de Gaulle et al (1992).

poorly documented. It is probable that the quality of postnatal nutrition influences the degree of statural catch-up. It is not surprising to see from recent studies in France (Thizon de Gaulle et al, 1992) and in Sweden (Albertsson-Wikland et al, 1993) that fewer than 10% of the infants will show a height inferior to the 2nd standard deviation under the average after the age of 2 years.

The production of GH by genetic engineering has led to its use for the treatment of severe growth retardations that are no longer linked to a deficit in GH (Turner syndrome, short stature and renal failure). The therapeutic trials carried out with GH on short statures due to IUGR gave favourable results. GH administration led to an important increase in the rate of growth with no particular side-effects and with no effect on glucose tolerance (Chatelain et al, 1994; Czernichow and Rappoport, 1993). Administered to pre-pubertal children for 3 years, GH allowed them to regain approximately 2 standard deviations. Although an acceleration of bone maturation was noted, the statural prognosis was improved by the end of the therapeutic period. However, the effect of high doses of GH (2–3 times the substitutive dose) on bone maturation should be closely examined. The evolution of growth rate at the end of the treatment remains to be studied and will be important in determining the statural prognosis of these children.

It is also probable that GH does not show the same efficacy in all types of small size related to IUGR. It has been shown, for instance, (Stanhope et al, 1991) that GH has limited efficacy in short stature due to the Silver-Russell syndrome. Finally, GH has metabolic effects in these children which may be beneficial and which must be borne in mind in any long-term evaluation. Thus, Leger et al (1994) were able to show that GH increased muscle mass in these children during the first few months of treatment and increased adipose mass after 2 years. These data, which should be confirmed in long-term studies, show a part of the beneficial effects of GH.

Adult height

Until recently, we only had available the results of sporadic studies carried out on small groups of young adults who had been born with IUGR. This work concluded that there was an average loss of 1 standard deviation with regard to the reference curves. A longitudinal study carried out in Sweden on 3650 infants born in the region of Göteborg (Albertsson-Wikland et al, 1993; Karlberg and Albertsson-Wikland, 1995) permitted the measurement of the adult height of 198 children (5.5%) born with weight or length inferior to 2 standard deviations below the average. At adulthood, 8% of this group still had a height inferior to −2 standard deviations, the statural prognosis being linked to the degree of statural retardation at birth.

The study also points out that this type of statural retardation represents 20% of the whole of the possible aetiologies of small size at the end of adolescence.

These studies showed how far-reaching IUGR is in terms of public health, and also the possible impact of GH on the statural prognosis of these children.

IUGR and metabolic problems

Two British surveys have indicated that low growth rates in utero are associated with high death rates from cardiovascular disease (Barker et al, 1993). Careful examination of men and women in different populations in Britain has shown that low weight at birth and low growth rate up to the age of 1 year are associated with increased blood pressure and increased plasma concentrations of glucose, pro-insulin, fibrinogen, factor VII and apolipoprotein B. These associations parallel those with death rates from cardiovascular diseases. Syndrome X, also known as insulin resistance syndrome, includes hypertension, glucose intolerance and dyslipidaemia. It has also been shown in the UK that low birthweight is a risk factor for syndrome X. This observation has been confirmed more recently by Valdez et al (1994) in a biethnic population in San Antonio, Texas, consisting of Mexican-Americans and non-Hispanic caucasians.

These observations have led to interesting hypotheses for the understanding of how fetal malnutrition is linked to abnormal function and disease in adult life, although no satisfactory explanations are presently available. Longitudinal studies of young adults born with IUGR will be important in future work to describe the natural history of syndrome X in this population. The possibility of early diagnosis will allow us to develop a prevention programme in this high risk population.

SUMMARY

The studies that have been carried out during the past 10 years on animals and in man have allowed us to progress in our understanding of the mechanisms underlying fetal growth in normal conditions and also in the fetus suffering from IUGR. Normal development of the fetus during the second half of gestation calls for harmonious co-operation between maternal, placental and fetal regulatory mechanisms. Any abnormality of these mechanisms will lead to fetal malnutrition and growth retardation. A central regulatory role is attributed to the growth factor IGF-I, which is present in all three compartments. Its level is lowered in the fetal compartment in cases of IUGR, and its value is rapidly normalized following birth and re-nutrition.

Children suffering from IUGR show a higher risk of mortality and morbidity than do normal children. Their postnatal growth is characterized by a catch-up growth period. Despite this, 8% of the subjects will have a small size as adults. Therapeutic trials with GH lead us to hope that an average growth retardation will be correctable by this method. Recent studies indicate that these children are at higher risk of cardiovascular complications, elevated blood pressure and non-insulin-dependent diabetes mellitus. The mechanisms that provoke these illnesses remain poorly understood but illustrate the complex modifications brought about by malnutrition in the uterus, and in the programming of illnesses in the adult.

REFERENCES

Albertsson-Wikland K, Wennergren G, Wennergren M et al (1993) Longitudinal follow-up of growth in children born small for gestational age. *Acta Paediatrica* **82:** 438–481.

Alsat E, Haziza J & Evain-Brion D (1993) Increase in epidermal growth factor receptor and its messenger ribonucleic acid levels with the differentiation of human trophoblast cells in culture. *Journal of Cellular Physiology* **154:** 122–128.

Baker J, Liu JP, Robertson EJ et al (1993) Role of insulin-like growth factors in embryonic and post-natal growth. *Cell* **75:** 73–82.

Barker DJP, Gluckman PD, Godfrey KM et al (1993) Fetal nutrition and cardiovascular disease in adult life. *Lancet* **341:** 938–941.

Beckers A, Stevenaert A, Foidart JM et al (1990) Placental and pituitary growth hormone secretion during pregnancy in acromegalic women. *Journal of Clinical Endocrinology and Metabolism* **71:** 725–731.

Chatelain P (1994) Dose-dependent catch-up growth after 2 years of growth hormone treatment in intrauterine growth-retarded children. *Journal of Clinical Endocrinology and Metabolism* **78:** 1454–1460.

Czernichow P & Rappoport R (1993) Growth hormone treatment of children with intrauterine growth retardation. In Muller EE, Cocchi D & Locatelli V (eds) *Growth Hormone and Somatomedins during Lifespan*, pp 161–170. Berlin: Springer-Verlag.

Davies DP (1981) Growth of small-for-dates babies. *Early Human Development* **5:** 95–105.

DeChiara TM, Efstratiadis A & Robertson EJ (1990) A growth-deficiency phenotype in heterozygous mice carrying an insulin-like growth factor II gene disrupted by targeting. *Nature* **345:** 78–80.

Evain-Brion D (1992) Growth factors and trophoblast differentiation. In Cedard L, Miller R & Firth A (eds) *Trophoblast Research*, pp 1–18. Rochester, Plenum Press.

Fitzhardinge PM & Inwood S (1989) Long-term growth in small-for-date children. *Acta Paediatrica Scandinavica* **349:** 27–33.

Fitzhardinge PM & Steven EM (1972) The small-for-date infant. I. Later growth patterns. *Pediatrics* **5:** 671–681.

Fondacci C, Alsat E, Gabriel R et al (1994) Alterations of human placental epidermal growth factor receptor in intrauterine growth retardation. *Journal of Clinical Investigation* **93:** 1149–1155.

Fowden AL, Hughes P & Comline RS (1989) The effect of insulin on the growth rate of the sheep fetus during late gestation. *Quarterly Journal of Experimental Physiology* **74:** 703–714.

Fancourt R, Campbell S, Harvey D et al (1976) Follow up study of small-for-dates babies. *British Medical Journal* **1:** 1453–1437.

Frankenne F, Closset J, Gomez F et al (1988) The physiology of growth hormones in pregnant women and partial characterization of the placental GH variant. *Journal of Clinical Endocrinology and Metabolism* **66:** 1171–1180.

Frankenne F, Scippo ML, Van Beeumen J et al (1990) Identification of placental human growth hormone as the GH-V gene expression product. *Journal of Clinical Endocrinology and Metabolism* **71:** 15–18.

Frankenne F, Alsat E, Scippo ML et al (1992) Evidence for the expression of growth hormone receptors in human placenta. *Biochemical and Biophysical Research Communications* **182:** 481–483.

Gabriel R, Alsat E & Evain-Brion D (1994) Alteration of epidermal growth factor receptor in placental membranes of smokers: relationship with intrauterine growth retardation. *American Journal of Obstetrics and Gynecology* **170:** 1238–1243.

Giudice LC, Irwin JC, Dsupin BA et al (1994) Insulin-like growth factors (IGFs), IGF binding proteins (IGFBPs) and IGFBP protease in human uterine endometrium: their potential relevance to endometrial cyclic function and maternal–embryonic interactions. In Baxter RC, Gluckman PD & Rosenfeld RG (eds) *The Insulin-like Growth Factors and their Regulatory Proteins*, pp 351–361. Amsterdam: Excerpta Medica.

Gluckman PD, Grumbach MM & Kaplan SL (1981) The neuroendocrine regulation and function of growth hormone and prolactin in the mammalian fetus. *Endocrine Reviews* **2:** 363–395.

Gluckman PD, Morel PCH, Ambler GR et al (1992a) Elevating maternal IGF-I in mice and rats alters the pattern of fetal growth by removing maternal constraint. *Journal of Endocrinology* **134:** R1–R3.

Gluckman PD, Gunn AJ, Wray A et al (1992b) Congenital idiopathic growth hormone deficiency associated with prenatal and early postnatal growth failures. *Journal of Pediatrics* **121:** 920–923.

Hill DJ, Riley SC, Basset T & Waters MJ (1992) Localization of the growth hormone receptor, identified by immunocytochemistry in 2nd trimester in human fetal tissues and in placenta throughout gestation. *Journal of Clinical Endocrinology and Metabolism* **75:** 646–650.

Honchliffe SA, Lynch MRJ, Sargant PH et al (1992) The effect of intrauterine growth retardation on the development of renal nephrons. *British Journal of Obstetrics and Gynaecology* **99:** 296–301.

Jones JI & Clemmons DR (1995) Insulin-like growth factors and their binding proteins: biological actions. *Endocrine Reviews* **16:** 3–34.

Karlberg J & Albertsson-Wikland K (1995) Growth in full-term small-for-gestational age infants: from birth to final height. *Pediatric Research* **38:** 733–739.

Koops BL (1978) Neurological sequelae in infants with intrauterine growth retardation. *Journal of Reproductive Medicine* **21:** 343–351.

Kroonsberg C, McCutcheon SN, Siddiqui RA et al (1989) Reproductive performance and fetal growth in female mice from lines divergently selected on the basis of plasma IGF-I concentrations. *Journal of Reproduction and Fertility* **87:** 349–353.

Lassare C, Hardouin S, Daffos F et al (1991) Serum insulin-like growth factors and insulin like growth factor binding proteins in the human fetus. Relationships with growth in normal subjects and in subjects with intrautrine growth retardation. *Pediatric Research* **29:** 219–225.

Leger J, Karel C, Legrand I et al (1994) Magnetic resonance imaging evaluation of adipose tissue and muscle tissue mass in children with growth hormone (GH) deficiency. Turner's syndrome and intrauterine growth retardation during the first year of treatment with GH. *Journal of Clinical Endocrinology and Metabolism* **78:** 904–909.

Leger J, Noel M, Limal JM & Czernichow P (1996a) Growth factors and intrauterine growth retardations II. Serum GH, IGF and IGFBP3 levels in children with intrauterine growth retardation as compared with normal controls: prospective study from birth to 2 years of age. *Pediatric Research* (in press).

Leger J, Oury JF, Noel M et al (1996b) Serum GH, IGF1, IGF2 and IGFBP3 levels in normally grown and growth retarded human fetuses during the second half of gestation. *Pediatric Research* (in press).

Lemons JA, Ridenour R & Orsini EN (1979) Congenital absence of the pancreas and intrauterine growth retardation. *Pediatrics* **64:** 255–257.

Liu JP, Baker J, Perkins S et al (1993) Mice carrying null mutations of the genes encoding insulin-like growth factor (IGF-1) and type 1 IGF receptor (IGF1r). *Cell* **75:** 59–72.

Merlet-Benichou C, Leroy B, Gilbert T et al (1993) Retard de croissance intra-utérin et déficit en nephrons. *Médecine et Science* **9:** 777–780.

Mirlesse V, Frankenne F, Alsat E et al (1993) Placental growth hormone levels in normal pregnancy and in pregnancies with intrauterine growth retardation. *Pediatric Research* **34:** 439–442.

Naeye RL, Blanc W & Paul C (1973) Effects of maternal nutrition on the human fetus. *Pediatrics* **52:** 494–503.

Oliver MH, Harding JE, Breier BH et al (1993) Glucose but not a mixed amino acid infusion regulates insulin-like growth factor-I concentrations in fetal sheep. *Pediatric Research* **34:** 62–65.

Ounsted M, Moar V & Scott A (1982) Growth in the first four years: diversity within groups of small-for-dates and large-for-dates babies. *Early Human Development* **7:** 29–39.

Ounsted M, Moar VA & Scott A (1989) Small for dates babies, gestational age and developmental ability at 7 years. *Early Human Development* **19:** 77–86.

Patel N, Alsat E, Igout A et al (1995) Glucose inhibits human placental GH secretion, in vitro. *Journal of Clinical Endocrinology and Metabolism* **80:** 1743–1746.

Scippo ML, Frankenne F, Hooghe-Peters EL et al (1992) Syncytiotrophoblastic localization of the human growth hormone variant mRNA in the placenta. *Molecular Cellular Endocrinology* **92:** R7–R13.

Stanhope R, Preece MA & Hamill G (1991) Does growth hormone treatment improve height attainment of children with intrauterine growth retardation? *Archives of Disease in Childhood* **66:** 1180–1183.

Tenovuo A, Kero P, Piekkala P et al (1987) Growth of 519 small for gestational age infants during the first two years of life. *Acta Paediatrica Scandinavica* **76:** 636–646.

Thizon de Gaulle I, Leger J & Czernichow P (1992) Retard de croissance intra-utérin: croissance postnatale et facteurs de croissance. In *Journées Parisiennes de Pédiatrie*, pp 63–70. Paris: Flammarion Medecine-Science.

Uzan M, Beaufils M, Breart G et al (1991) Prevention of fetal growth retardation with low dose aspirin: findings of the EPREDA trial. *Lancet* **337:** 1427–1431.

Valdez R, Atens MA, Bradshaw BS & Stern MP (1994) Birth weight and adult health outcomes in a biethnic US population. *Diabetology* **37:** 624–663.
Zegher F De, Bettendorf M, Kaplan SL & Grumbach SM (1988) Hormone ontogeny in the ovine fetus. XXI. The effect of insulin-like growth factor-I on plasma fetal growth-hormone, insulin and glucose concentrations. *Endocrinology* **123:** 658–660.

3

Screening for congenital hypothyroidism: effectiveness and clinical outcome

ANNETTE GRÜTERS

Congenital hypothyroidism is known to be one of the most common causes of preventable mental retardation in children. Since it had been evident from studies of the mental development in patients detected by clinical symptoms that early treatment in the first weeks of life resulted in a better intellectual and neurological outcome (Klein et al, 1972), mass newborn screening was introduced as early as 20 years ago in some European countries as well as in Canada and the USA (Dussault et al, 1975; Illig and Rodriguez, 1976).

When evaluating the results that have been achieved by newborn screening, the following crucial questions have to be answered:

1. Is neonatal screening necessary or have symptoms in the first weeks of life led to the diagnosis in a significant number of newborns before the screening result was available?
2. Which screening strategies are effective and should therefore be recommended?
3. What is the prevalence and aetiology of the different forms of congenital hypothyroidism?
4. What are the reasons for missing the diagnosis in neonatal screening?
5. What is the outcome of the patients with early diagnosis and treatment?

CLINICAL SYMPTOMS OF PATIENTS DETECTED BY NEONATAL SCREENING

Soon after the introduction of the first screening programmes, it became clear that a significant number of newborns already had clinical symptoms at the age of 3 weeks, which was the usual time for the first presentation of newborns with a positive screening result during the first years of most of the screening programmes. When scores were calculated by comparing babies with clinical symptoms with matched healthy controls, significant higher scores in the hypothyroid newborns were found (Letarte et al, 1981), and these symptoms were more prevalent in newborns with lower thyroid hormone levels at diagnosis. In this respect especially, the finding of a

Baillière's Clinical Paediatrics —
Vol. 4, No. 2, May 1996
ISBN 0–7020–2180–6
0963–6714/96/020259 + 18 $12.00/00

delayed bone maturation, which can be investigated by X-ray of the knee and ankle and more recently also by ultrasound studies (Bassir et al, 1995), is significantly correlated with the more severe forms of congenital hypo-thyroidism and allows the estimation of the onset of fetal hypothyroidism (Glorieux et al, 1992). It was speculated that by using such a clinical neonatal hypothyroid index—similar to the performance of Apgar scores—the most severely affected newborns would certainly be clinically detectable before the development of gross signs and symptoms developed (Letarte et al, 1981). The presence of clinical symptoms in the first weeks of life is not surprising, since it has become more evident from recent research that thyroid hormone receptors are present very early during mammalian development. It has been shown that thyroid hormones play an important role during fetal development (Stein et al, 1989; Calvo et al, 1990; Contempre et al, 1993), especially through the regulation of the expression of several genes in the developing nervous system, for example RC3 (neurogranin) (Bernal and Pekonen, 1984), tubulin (Stein et al, 1989), and NGFI-A (Pipanon et al, 1992). The recently reported maternal–fetal thyroid hormone transfer in animal models and the human seems to protect the hypothyroid fetus to a certain extent from the adverse effects of the fetal thyroid hormone deficiency, and therefore early treatment might be able completely to reverse the effects in the majority of the patients. However, in patients with severe fetal hypothyroidism (e.g. due to athyreosis) in combination with maternal hypothyroxinaemia (e.g. due to iodine deficiency), the potential risk of irreversible sequelae of fetal hypothyroidism has to be considered.

Indeed, the appearance of many newborns with congenital hypo-thyroidism apparent in the first weeks of life is strikingly typical of those with the disease discovered later (Figure 1). The question of how many of the newborns detected by neonatal screening give rise to a clinical suspicion of congenital hypothyroidism before the screening result is available has not been addressed in the reports that have been published. In

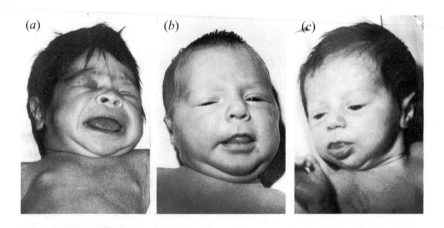

Figure 1. Three patients with congenital hypothyroidism at 8–10 days of life.

our experience of 120 newborns with congenital hypothyroidism who presented with a mean age of 8 days (range 5–12 days) symptoms were detectable in a considerable number of patients by the paediatrician who examined the infant because of a suspicious screening result (Table 1). However, in none of these newborns had the clinical suspicion of congenital hypothyroidism been raised before, although on the 4–6th day of life all of them were carefully examined by a paediatrician as part of Germany's routine neonatal care programme.

Therefore it can be concluded that mild symptoms of neonatal hypothyroidism are present as early as the first 2 weeks of life, owing to the dependancy of the fetal development on thyroid hormones, but that they escape detection during routine paediatric investigation, so biochemical screening is therefore the only effective tool for early diagnosis. Careful follow-up of all patients is mandatory since the reversibility of these symptoms is clearly dependent on a rapid normalization of thyroid function.

Table 1. Symptoms of permanent and transient congenital hypothyroidism in newborns with congenital hypothyroidism at first presentation because of an increased TSH-level on neonatal screening. (The investigator was aware of the screening result but not of the definitive diagnosis.)

Symptom	Permanent ($N = 92$)	Transient ($N = 28$)
Open posterior fontanelle	63	2
Hyperbilirubinaemia	57	8
Mottled skin	37	2
Poor feeding	36	1
Enlarged tongue	34	1
Umbilical hernia	31	2
Typical face	30	0
Muscular hypotonia	27	1
Obstipation	2	0
Bradycardia	1	0
Hypothermia	1	0
Respiratory distress syndrome	1	0
Delayed bone age	68	2

SCREENING STRATEGIES

The first mass screening programmes in North America and Japan were established by using the determination of T4 in dried filter paper blood spots of the fifth day of life (Dussault et al, 1975). However other American screening centres already at that time preferred the determination of thyroid-stimulating hormone (TSH) in cord blood (Walfish et al, 1979). In almost all European countries, TSH was the screening parameter of choice from the beginning (Illig and Rodriguez, 1976). The argument in favour of using T4 as the primary test, usually followed by a determination of TSH in any screening specimen with a low T4, is the ability to detect infants with hypothalamic–hypopituitary hypothyroidism, thyroxine-binding globulin (TBG) deficiency and thyroid hormone resistance. However, the major disadvantages of this procedure are the risk of missing newborns with compensated hypothyroidism with normal T4 levels (but usually already increased TSH levels) due to large ectopic glands or milder defects of thyroid hormone biosynthesis, and the high frequency of low T4 levels in premature and ill newborns, which will lead to an increased number of control investigations. The frequency of primary congenital hypothyroidism in countries using T4 as the primary screening parameter—1 in 5000–8000 newborns—is therefore lower than the prevalence of 1 in 3000–4000 in the programmes using as the primary approach TSH determination (Toublanc, 1992), which will detect also patients with subclinical hypothyroidism and already elevated TSH levels. It can be questioned whether it is necessary to detect at birth these milder forms of congenital hypothyroidism, which have presented before screening probably as juvenile acquired hypothyroidism. Therefore the reason that is most strongly in favour of using TSH as the primary screening approach is the significantly lower rate of control investigations.

The number of elevated TSH levels in a newborn population is clearly dependent on the iodine supply, with an increased rate of concentration above the usual recall limits of 15–20 mU/l in regions with significant iodine deficiency (Delange et al, 1989). Therefore TSH screening is also suitable to monitor the iodine supply of a newborn population. This was observed even within the re-unified city of Berlin, where high TSH levels were more prevalent in the former Western parts lacking a sufficient iodine supply compared with the former Eastern part, where a nationwide iodization programme was effective (Grüters et al, 1995). Interestingly, some of the North American screening centres have recently switched to strategies with a primary TSH determination.

Factors that have more impact on the effectiveness of screening programmes for congenital hypothyroidism than the screening method itself are those related to the management of the programme. Guidelines for screening programmes for congenital hypothyroidism have recently been published by the American Academy of Pediatrics (1993) and the European Society for Pediatric Endocrinology (Grüters et al, 1993) (Table 2).

A prerequisite for the effectiveness of a mass screening is the coverage of close to 100% of all newborns of a region, which has been achieved in most but clearly not all of the Western European countries. To achieve close to 100% coverage, screening for congenital hypothyroidism should be coupled to the screening for other metabolic diseases and should be centralized. The work-up of newborns with a pathological screening result should include the determination of serum TSH and free (T4) levels, and the initiation of therapy should be performed in collaboration with a paediatric endocrinologist to avoid unnecessarily long-term treatment periods in patients with transient forms of congenital hypothyroidism. For high sensitivity (ability to detect all affected newborns) and specificity (decreased by false positive results), the time at which the blood sample is taken is a crucial factor.

Table 2. Guidelines for screening programmes for congenital hypothyroidism of the European Society for Paediatric Endocrinology.

- Combination with screening for metabolic diseases
- Centralized laboratories covering at least 40 000 births
- Confirmatory tests: TSH and T4 or fT4 in serum
- Responsibility of screening centre for the follow-up of positive results until congenital hypothyroidism is proven or disproven
- Screening method of choice: TSH in blood spots by sensitive measurement
- Sampling not after the 5th day of life; earlier sampling possible
- A second sample should be taken from premature infants, sick newborns in intensive care (especially after exchange transfusion and dopamine treatment) and after iodine overload
- Treatment of choice: l-thyroxine (10–15 µg/kg per day)
- Reconfirmation of diagnosis at 2 years of life by TSH, T4, TG, ultrasound and approach of definitive diagnosis

TSH values are slightly higher in serum from the cord than in that of later life. During the first 6 hours after birth, levels rise abruptly to very high values, and they then decline over the next 24–36 hours (Foley et al, 1994). Subsequent to the TSH surge, T4 levels peak around 24 hours of life and then also gradually decrease over the next few days. In recent years, the more frequent early discharge of mothers and newborns from maternity wards has made consideration of the time of specimen collection necessary. Since many current TSH screening methods use monoclonal antibodies, reliable results can already be obtained after 24 hours of life, because the TSH concentrations will have declined to values below the recall limits. (Dussault and Morrisette, 1993; Dussault et al, 1994). Therefore no significant increase in the frequency of control investigations has to be anticipated when screening samples are collected any time after the first day of life and sensitive assays are used. TSH screening for congenital hypothyroidism is also possible in cord blood. It is advisable to test every infant before discharge from the nursery regardless of the time of discharge, because the use of age-adjusted cut-off levels for TSH (Dussault and Morrisette, 1993) enables reliable screening at any age. So far, all screening centres recommend a second specimen if the first was collected within the first 24 hours. If the screening sample is not taken in the maternity ward, the initiation of the screening test will depend on the mother's ability to understand and accept the importance of this preventive medical care.

PREVALENCE OF CONGENITAL HYPOTHYROIDISM

The incidence of congenital hypothyroidism in different parts of the world is comparable, ranging from 1 in 3000 to 1 in 4000 newborns (Toublanc, 1992). There is no significant seasonal variation, but there is some evidence that the ethnic background plays a role, because of the observation of an increased incidence in hispanic newborns and a decreased frequency in the black population (Brown et al, 1981). Mass newborn screening is only established in the Western European countries, North America, Japan, New

Zealand, Australia and some South American countries, such as Brazil, Chile and Equador, but the incidence of congenital hypothyroidism is still unknown in many parts of the world, including Eastern Europe and Africa. In some Eastern European countries, screening programmes were established with the help of Western countries, for example in Bulgaria with the help of Switzerland. Before more efforts can be made to establish screening for congenital hypothyroidism in all parts of the world, it has to be ensured first that proper substitution of thyroid hormone can be guaranteed, since l-thyroxine preparations are so far not available in most third world countries and also parts of the former Soviet Union.

In view of the possible influences of ethnic background and iodine nutrition on the prevalence of congenital hypothyroidism, it is astonishing that the incidence is so uniform (Toublanc, 1992). The worldwide distribution for the different forms of permanent congenital hypothyroidism is also surprisingly similar, 80–85% resulting from different variants of thyroid dysgenesis (athyreosis, ectopy or hypoplasia) and 15–20% resulting from assumed defects of thyroid hormone biosynthesis (Toublanc, 1990a). It has been noted above that the almost doubled incidence of patients with congenital hypothyroidism detected through newborn screening,

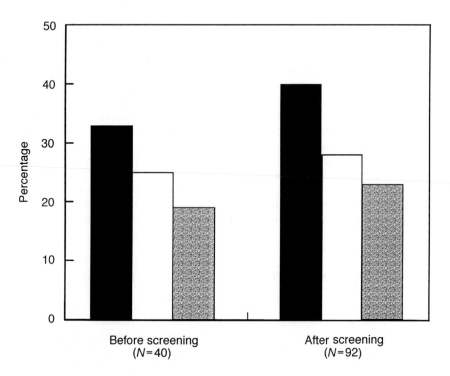

Figure 2. Frequencies of the different types of congenital hypothyroidism before and after the introduction of neonatal screening in Berlin. (■) Athyrosis; (☐) Ectopy; (▨) Thyroid present.

compared with the incidence of patients previously detected by clinical symptoms, might be due to a higher incidence of patients with compensated neonatal thyroid hypothyroidism due to large ectopic glands or milder defects of biosynthesis. Few data are available regarding the frequencies of the more and less severe forms. In our own groups of patients diagnosed clinically before or after the introduction of newborn screening, the distribution of the different types of congenital hypothyroidism was similar (Figure 2), indicating that the difference in the total frequencies cannot be explained only by the detection of milder forms through screening, but that a significant number of severe cases failed to be diagnosed on clinical grounds before screening programmes were introduced (Alm et al, 1984).

AETIOLOGY OF CONGENITAL HYPOTHYROIDISM

The different forms of congenital hypothyroidism (Table 3) occur sporadically; familial cases are rare. Congenital hypothyroidism due to thyroid dysgenesis is 2–3 times more frequent in girls than in boys, and the aetiology is still unknown. Research into germ-line or somatic mutations of genes for thyroid-specific proteins, such as the TSH receptor, or of thyroid-specific transcription factors may give new insight into the pathogenesis of these malformations. In some mothers of newborns with thyroid dysgenesis, growth-blocking or cytotoxic antibodies have been identified (Bogner et al, 1989; van der Gaag et al, 1985), but it remains necessary to study whether these antibodies are the cause of congenital hypothyroidism or the consequence of a defect of the fetal thyroid gland, because the frequency of autoimmune thyroid disease in mothers of patients with congenital hypothyroidism is in general not increased.

In contrast, patients with an eutopic gland are equally sex distributed, as could be expected for the assumed defects of thyroid hormone biosynthesis, which are inherited as an autosomal recessive trait. However, the frequencies of the different possible defects of biosynthesis are unknown, although moleular genetic studies are now possible at least for mutations of the TPO and thyroglobulin gene, for which mutations have been identified

Table 3. Differential diagnosis of congenital hypothyroidism.

Permanent hypothyroidism	Transient hypothyroidism
(1:3000)	(1:8500)
1. Thyroid dysgenesis (85%)	1. Maternal or neonatal exposure to iodide (> 90%)
Athyreosis (40%)	PVC-iodine (> 90%)
Ectopy (30%)	Contrast media
Hypoplasia (5%)	Kaliumjodatum
	Amiodarone
2. Dyshormonogenesis (15%)	2. Maternal TSH receptor-blocking antibodies (5%)
3. Thyroid hormone resistance	3. Maternal anti-thyroid drug therapy
4. TRH or TSH deficiency	4. Iodine deficiency

in familial cases (Bikker et al, 1995). It is important to clarify the molecular basis of these defects in the near future, not only from a research point of view, but also for the sake of the individual patient. In contrast to the mentally retarded patients discovered before screening was available, the patients detected through screening will reproduce normally, so there is more need for genetic counselling. Therefore a definitive diagnosis and clarification of the aetiology should be approached in all patients as early as possible (Figure 3).

Thyroid imaging plays a key role in the differential diagnostic work-up. However, in contrast to former reports (Delange, 1989), routine scanning is no longer recommended, especially not in the newborn, because there is a significant number of unreliable results, particularly when these studies are performed by inexperienced investigators. In addition, false scanning results were obtained in newborns due to maternal blocking immuno-globulins or perinatal iodine contamination (Connors and Styne, 1986). Ultrasound studies can reveal whether thyroid tissue is already present in the normal position in the newborn period. If no thyroid gland is detectable by ultrasound, the differential diagnosis between athyreosis and ectopy can be made by taking into account the thyroxine and thyreoglobulin concentrations and the bone age. If thyroxine and thyreoglobulin levels are measurable and bone age is not delayed, it can be assumed that the rest of thyroid tissue is present in an ectopic position. Furthermore, the knowledge

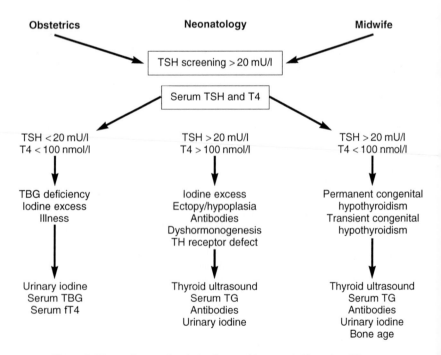

Figure 3. Diagnostic procedure in newborns with congenital hypothyroidism.

of the severity of the disease as assessed by the T4 level at diagnosis is more important for the prognosis and will have an impact on the therapeutic management of the individual patient.

A number of newborns with elevated TSH levels in neonatal screening will have transient hypothyroidism or hyperthyreotrophinaemia. In the majority of these patients, the TSH and T4 concentrations will be normalized when confirmatory tests are performed within the first 3 weeks of life. Transient hypothyroidism can result from maternal anti-thyroid antibodies (Matsuura et al, 1980), endemic iodine deficiency or perinatal exposure to iodine excess. In Berlin, perinatal iodine contamination owing to the use of povidone iodine is the most frequent cause of hyperthyreotropinaemia (Grüters et al, 1983), and postnatal iodine exposure during intensive care accounts for the increased frequency of transient hypothyroidism in premature newborns (l'Allemand et al, 1987). Transient hypothyroidism is a rare condition, ranging from 1 in 8000 newborns in Europe to 1 in 50 000 newborns in North America; the incidence of transient hyperthyreotropin-aemia is quite variable (0.01–0.8%) and depends on the frequency of iodine excess and the nutritional iodine supply in the population (Delange et al, 1978, 1989; Grüters et al, 1995).

REASONS FOR MISSING THE DIAGNOSIS IN NEONATAL SCREENING FOR CONGENITAL HYPOTHYROIDISM

The frequencies of missed cases and the reasons for missing the diagnosis depend on the type of screening strategy. As mentioned above, the lower incidence of congenital hypothyroidism in screening approaches using T4 as the primary test results from missing patients with compensated forms of congenital hypothyroidism, when thyroxine levels are normal or borderline because of the residual function of either ectopic or eutopic thyroid tissue.

In North America, some states therefore introduced a second test at 2–6 weeks of age (American Academy of Pediatrics, 1993), and this revealed that 10% of the patients would have been missed by T4 screening alone. Most of these infants were less severely affected and would have gone undiagnosed until an age when they would have been falsely classified as acquired hypothyroidism. Some of them already had acquired transient hypothyroidism due to iodine overload in the first weeks of life. The risk of missing these patients is lower in screening programmes using cut-off limits of T4 in the lower normal range (10th percentile) and additional TSH tests in all those newborns with low T4 tests. In one simultaneous screening of TSH and T4 in almost 100 000 newborns in Quebec, only one patient would have been missed by T4 screening alone.

Using TSH as the primary screening approach, patients with hypothalamic–pituitary hypothyroidism (1 in 10 000 newborns) will be missed. Since these newborns do not usually have isolated TRH or TSH deficiencies but instead multiple pituitary hormone deficiencies, including those of ACTH and growth hormone, they are at risk of irreversible damage from unnoticed periods of hypoglycaemia. Also, patients with thyroid hormone resistance will be missed by TSH screening alone. Since it is now evident that not only the patients with general resistance (GTHR) but also those with milder defects may suffer from longstanding neurological, auditory and attention deficit problems, it might be worthwhile aiming at an early detection by neonatal screening (Refetoff et al, 1993).

Furthermore, there is some evidence that some infants with congenital hypothyroidism due to thyroid dysgenesis are born with low or normal T4 concentrations and TSH levels below the most commonly used recall limit of 20 mU/l whole blood or 40 mU/l serum. Serum TSH levels increase during the first weeks of life and are then typical for primary hypothyroidism (Harada et al, 1995). The reasons for this remain unclear. Some of these screening assays had a poor reproducibility, so that re-testing of levels just below 20 mU/l had to be performed in 5% of all newborns, and it was concluded that the recall limit in these assays ought to be lowered to 10 mU/l. Using sensitive radio-immuno- or immunofluorescent TSH assays with a cut-off of 20 mU/l, we only have missed one patient with a low TSH screening result of 18 mU/l, who had developed symptoms of hypothyroidism and a TSH of over 200 mU/l at 18 months of age. In this girl, hypothyroidism was due to a deiodinase defect and was masked in the newborn screening by prenatal exposure to povidone iodine (Grüters et al, 1994). In the Quebec study 2 in 100 000 newborns would have been missed by primary TSH screening (Dussault and Morrisette, 1983).

More frequent reasons for failed diagnosis from either screening approach are missing or insufficient samples, human errors in processing the samples or erroneously reported results. In Germany from 1981 to 1991, 36 newborns were missed for these reasons, and some were severely handicapped. Insufficient and unsaturated blood spots will result in TSH levels that are too low, as will diluting the blood spots with spilled fluids. When using immunofluorescent techniques for TSH determination (Delfia), EDTA blood (spotted on filter paper with EDTA-coated capillaries) will lead to falsely low levels.

The diagnosis will also be missed if the sample is collected after a blood transfusion, exchange transfusion or feto-fetal transfusion (de Zegher and Vanderschueren-Lodewyckx, 1989) or during dopamine treatment. In preterms, a second specimen should be collected at an age corresponding to 36 weeks gestation, because at screening TSH levels might have been low, despite primary hypothyroidism, because of hypothalamic immaturity or critical illness. The issue of whether the transient hypothyroxinaemia without TSH elevation in the premature infant is a condition that should be treated with l-thyroxine is still controversial. Few longitudinal studies of the development of these children that have controlled for the many confounding factors that influence the outcome of premature infants are so far available (Chowdry et al, 1984). Infants of mothers with Graves' disease may have received maternal polyclonal antibodies, and development of hypothyroidism due to blocking antibodies can be delayed when stimulating antibodies predominate in the first weeks of life.

Because there are many possible reasons for missing the diagnosis in neonatal screening (Table 4), physicians and especially paediatricians

Table 4. Reasons for missing the diagnosis with different screening strategies.

- Compensated hypothyroidism due to large ectopic glands or mild defects of biosynthesis
- Prematurity or severe illness
- Masking of defects of biosynthesis leading to iodine deficiency by perinatal iodine exposure
- Transfusion, exchange transfusion or feto–fetal transfusion
- Dopamine treatment
- Maternal anti-thyroid drugs
- Insufficient or contaminated samples
- Error in processing the sample or reporting the result.

should therefore still be aware of the clinical picture of congenital hypothyroidism in early life, and they should not hesitate to initiate thyroid function tests in any infant in whom they suspect hypothyroidism, even in the face of a normal newborn screening result.

OUTCOME OF THE PATIENTS WITH EARLY DIAGNOSIS AND TREATMENT OF CONGENITAL HYPOTHYROIDISM

All published reports which compared the outcome of patients with an early diagnosis and treatment of congenital hypothyroidism with matched controls or siblings have shown that the mean IQs of these patients have normalized. However, in some of the studies, significant differences of 2–11 IQ points in the full or verbal IQs, compared with normal controls, have been documented (Table 5). Therefore it is important to investigate which medical or social factors might influence the outcome, in order to minimize their negative influence through treatment or follow-up strategies.

Table 5. IQ findings in children with early treated congenital hypothyroidism, compared with controls.

Study	Year	Country	N	IQ of hypothyroid patients	IQ of controls
New England Congenital Hypothyroidism Collaborative	1985	USA	72	106	109
Glorieux	1985	Canada	36	102	106
Tillotson et al	1994	France	49	116	118
Heyerdahl et al	1991	Norway	27	88	99
Illicki and Larsson	1991	Sweden	24	105	105
Rovet	1992	Canada	95	107	114
Kooistra et al	1994	Netherlands	62	97	103
Tillotson et al	1994	UK	344	105	112

Age at onset of treatment

In all newborns in whom the diagnosis of congenital hypothyroidism has been confirmed by the determination of the serum (free) T4, T3 and TSH concentrations, and in those in whom test results of control investigations will not be obtained within 24 hours, immediate l-thyroxine substitution should be initiated, because it has been shown that, especially in the more severe forms of congenital hypothyroidism (Glorieux et al, 1988), an earlier onset of treatment is associated with a better outcome (Illig et al, 1987; Fuggle et al, 1991). However, some other studies did not find an effect of the age at start of the treatment on the outcome (Kooistra et al, 1994; Tillotson et al, 1994), probably because the range of the age at onset of treatment has narrowed in most of the screening programmes with improved screening and recall procedures. Moreover, treatment is usually more delayed in those patients with close to normal T4 levels at diagnosis, because in these patients a transient form was first ruled out before therapy was started, and most of the studies correlating outcome and onset of treatment have not taken this into account.

Initial l-thyroxine dose

The optimal starting dose for correcting congenital hypothyroidism is still controversial. Earlier studies suggested that a fixed dose of 6–8 µg thyroxine/kg would be sufficient, because with this dose T4 and T3 levels within the euthyroid range were obtained in a reasonable time (Abassi and Aldige, 1977; Rezvani and DiGeorge, 1977). Follow-up studies then indicated that these doses might not be sufficient to normalize mental development in all patients (Dubuis et al, 1994), and in one study the better results compared with other studies were related to a more rapid correction of T4 levels (Mitchell et al, 1989). Therefore, current guidelines (Fisher and Foley, 1989; American Academy of Pediatrics, 1993; Grüters et al, 1993) recommend higher initial doses (10–15 µg/kg per day) to reduce the period of postnatal hypothyroidism by achieving a more rapid normalization not only of T4, but also of TSH levels. Comparing two groups of patients with a high (> 7.8 µg/kg per day) and low (< 7.8 µg/kg per day) initial dose, a recent study showed that full-scale IQ and verbal IQ, as well as several sub-test results, were significantly better in the high-dose group (Rovet and Ehrlich, 1995). However, this study was retrospective, not randomized and there was a significantly earlier onset of treatment in the high-dose group. In a subgroup of 9 of our patients treated with a lower dose of 6–9 µg/kg per day, compared with the patients receiving the commonly used higher dose of 10–14 µg/kg per day, no significant difference in full-scale IQ was found in spite of a significantly later normalization of TSH levels. Also, other studies were not able to detect an influence of the initial dose, but again these studies were not prospective and lower doses might have been used intentionally in the patients with less severe types of congenital hypothyroidism. With common tests to investigate behaviour in children with chronic illnesses, behavioural problems were found in the initially high-dose group in a recent publication (Rovet and Ehrlich, 1995), but at the age of 7 and 8 years, when testing was done, the former high-dose group received lower l-thyroxine doses, leading to lower circulating thyroid hormone levels. Therefore the authors mentioned that the negative association of starting dose and behaviour should be interpreted with caution. Prospective studies are warranted to investigate the optimal dose at onset of therapy.

Compliance

Earlier studies have already indicated that an impaired outcome despite early treatment is associated with poor compliance with therapy (New England Congenital Hypothyroidism Collaborative, 1985). More recent studies have also confirmed this by correlating mean thyroxine levels during treatment or the frequency of TSH elevations to outcome in terms of IQ (New England Congenital Hypothyroidism Collaborative, 1990; Toublanc, 1990b; Heyerdahl et al, 1991). Since compliance is dependent on the ability of the parents to understand and accept the necessity of treatment, it is not surprising that the socio-economic environment has a significant impact on the outcome (Toublanc, 1990b; Simons et al, 1994; Tillotson et al, 1994).

Severity of congenital hypothyroidism

The severity of hypothyroidism at birth is characterized by the thyroid hormone levels at diagnosis and the symptoms of hypothyroidism that are present, most objectively by the assessment of skeletal maturation. The type of hypothyroidism (athyreosis, ectopy, hypoplasia or hypofunction of the normally sited gland) cannot be defined unequivocally by thyroid imaging in each case, and therefore some studies were not able to find an influence of the type of diagnosis on the outcome (Virtanen et al, 1989). Although there is a significant difference between the groups of patients with athyreosis and ectopy concerning the mean TSH and T4 levels at diagnosis, there is a wide overlap, so that the severity in terms of hypofunction might not correlate to the type of hypothyroidism in the individual patient (Figure 4).

Deficits of development could be correlated to a delayed bone age in many (Rochiccioli et al, 1984; Rovet et al, 1987; Glorieux et al, 1988; Virtanen et al, 1989), but not all (Illicki and Larsson, 1991), studies. A more precise description of the severity may be obtained by the T4 levels at diagnosis: a low thyroxine level (< 30 or 40 nmol/l) was related to a deficit of mental development in most of the studies (Glorieux, 1988; Rovet et al, 1987; Fuggle, 1994). A conclusive assessment was published from a large cohort of patients ($N = 361$ and 315 controls) in the UK (Tillotson et al, 1994). In this study, a discontinuous effect of the severity of congenital hypothyroidism on mental development was demonstrated, with a risk of having a 10 point deficit in IQ with a thyroxine level of less than 40 nmol/l. The assignment to the group of patients of a lower social class accounted for another 10 point decrease in IQ. Surprisingly, although the onset of treatment varied considerably from 1 to 173 days, no obvious effect of a later onset on mental development was observed. The authors concluded that even after early diagnosis and treatment, the intrauterine hypothyroidism of the more severe cases has an appreciable effect on intellectual development, and that the maternal transfer of thyroid hormone

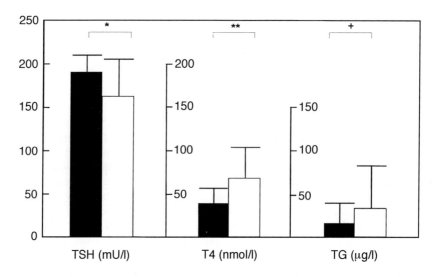

Figure 4. TSH, T4 and TG levels at diagnosis in newborns with congenital hypothyroidism (mean/SD). * $P < 0.02$; ** $P < 0.002$; + Not significant. (▪) Athyrosis; (☐) Ectopy.

to the hypothyroid fetus (Vulsma et al, 1989) is insufficient to protect the fetus if hypothyroidism is severe.

Some studies were not able to demonstrate this relationship between severity of congenital hypothyroidism and outcome (New England Congenital Hypothyroidism Collaborative, 1985; Illicki and Larsson, 1991). Also, in our patients, there was no difference in the IQ of patients with a T4 less than or greater than 32 nmol/l at diagnosis. However, as in Illicki's study, the onset of treatment in our patients was very early, with a median of 8 (range 5–21) days. Therefore it may be speculated that a very early onset of treatment might be able to rescue fetal impairment.

SUMMARY

It is now clear that screening for congenital hypothyroidism is the only tool to detect this condition within the early neonatal period. Cost-effective TSH screening is the procedure of choice any time after the first 24 hours, although some cases would be detected only by a combined TSH/T4 (fT4) screening approach.

There is evidence that there is a threshold effect for the severity of congenital hypothyroidism on the outcome, and therefore the benefits that can be achieved by early treatment will probably be to some extent limited. However, no study so far has been controlled for all important variables, such as socio-economic score, compliance, onset of treatment and initial l-thyroxine dose, that have been shown to have an influence on mental development (Table 6).

Table 6. Factors that have been shown to influence the outcome of early treated congenital hypothyroidism.

- Onset of treatment
- Dose of l-thyroxine
- Severity of congenital hypothyroidism
  —different forms of congenital hypothyroidism
  —T4 level at diagnosis
  —bone age at diagnosis
- Socio-economic score (SES)
- Compliance

For routine practice, it is advisable to aim for a rapid normalization of thyroid function parameters by using a dose of 10–15 µg/kg per day, especially in the more severely affected newborns, as assessed by the determination of thyroid hormone levels and the bone age. During the first weeks of treatment, the dose should therefore be individualized and treatment frequently and carefully monitored to minimize residual fetal impairment and avoid behavioural problems. Although concern has been raised in the UK study (Tillotson et al, 1994) that up to 10% of children will still need special education, other studies have shown a normal school performance regardless of severity (New England Congenital Hypothyroidism Collaborative, 1990). Therefore it can be concluded that even if mild deficits are still present in some patients, the normal school performance of most patients has proven that neonatal screening for congenital hypothyroidism is one of the major achievements of preventive paediatric medicine. Further improvement of this achievement will be possible through optimization of screening strategies and therapy.

REFERENCES

Abassi V & Aldige C (1977) Evaluation of sodium L-thyroxine requirement in replacement therapy of hypothyroidism. *Journal of Pediatrics* **90:** 291–295.

Alm J, Hagenfeld L, Larsson A & Lundberg K (1984) Incidence of congenital hypothyroidism: retrospective study of neonatal laboratory screening versus clinical symptoms as indicator leading to diagnosis. *British Medical Journal* **298:** 1171–1175.

American Academy of Pediatrics (1993) Newborn screening for congenital hypothyroidism: recommended guidelines. *Pediatrics* **91:** 1203–1209.

Bernal J & Pekonen F (1984) Ontogenesis of the nuclear 3,5,3′-triiodothyronine receptor in the human fetal brain. *Endocrinology* **114:** 677–679.

Bassir C, Bührer C & Grüters A (1995) Skelettreifebestimmung mit Sonografie von Knie und Fuß bei gesunden Neugeborenen und Neugeborenen mit angeborener Hypothyreose. *Monatsschrift Kinderheilkunde* **143:** 179.

Bikker H, Vulsma T, Baas F & de Vijlder JJM (1995) Identification of five novel inactivating mutations in the human thyroid peroxidase gene by denaturing gradient gel electrophoresis. *Human Mutations* **6:** 9–16.

Bogner U, Grüters A, Sigle B et al (1989) Cytotoxic antibodies in congenital hypothyroidism. *Journal of Clinical Endocrinology and Metabolism* **68:** 671–675.

Brown AL, Fernhoff PM, Milner J et al (1981) Racial differences in the birth prevalence of congenital hypothyroidism. *Journal of Pediatrics* **99:** 934–936.

Calvo R, Obregon MJ, Ruiz de Ona C et al (1990) Congenital hypothyroidism, as studied in rats. Crucial role of maternal thyroxine but not on 3,5,3′-triiodothyronine in the protection of the fetal brain. *Journal of Clinical Investigation* **86:** 889–899.

Chowdry P, Scanlon JW & Auerbach R (1984) Results of controlled double blind study of thyroid replacement in very low birth weight premature infants with hypothyroxinemia. *Pediatrics* **73:** 301–305.

Connors M & Styne D (1986) Transient neonatal athyreosis resulting from thyrotropin binding inhibitory immunoglobulins. *Pediatrics* **78:** 278–281.

Contempre B, Calvo R, Jauniaux E et al (1993) Thyroid hormones in human embryonic cavities during the first trimester of gestation. *Journal of Endocrinological Investigation* **16 (supplement 2):** 56–63.

Delange F (1989) Iodine nutrition and hypothyoidism. In Delange F, Fischer DA & Glinoer D (eds) *Research in Congenital Hypothroidism,* pp 173–182. New York: Plenum Press.

Delange F, Dodion J, Wolter R et al (1978) Transient hypothyroidism in the newborn infant. *Journal of Pediatrics* **92:** 974–978.

Delange F, de Vijlder J, Morreale de Escobar G et al (1989) Significance of early diagnostic data in congenital hypothyroidism: report of the subcommittee on neonatal hypothroidism of the European Thyroid Association. In Delange F, Fischer DA & Glinoer D (eds) *Research in Congenital Hypothroidism,* pp 225–231.

Dubuis JM, Richer F, Glorieux J et al (1994) Should all patients with congenital hypothyroidism (CH) be treated with 10–15 µg/kg/day of levothyroxine (T4)? *Pediatric Research* **80:** 745–749.

Dussault JH & Morrisette J (1983) Higher sensitivity of primary thyrotropin in screening for congenital hypothyroidism: a myth? *Journal of Clinical Endocrinology and Metabolism* **56:** 849–853.

Dussault JH & Morrisette J (1993) Analysis of TSH levels measured by a screening program in regard of the day of sampling. *Abstracts of the 2nd Meeting of the International Society of Newborn Screening,* Lille, p 73.

Dussault JH, Grenier A, Morrisette J & Mitchell M (1994) Filterpaper TSH levels in the first 24 hours of life. *Abstracts of the 10th National Screening Symposium,* Seattle, p 27.

Dussault JH, Coulombe P, Laberge C et al (1975) Preliminary report on a mass screening program for neonatal hypothyroidism. *Journal of Pediatrics* **86:** 670–674.

Fisher DA & Foley B (1989) Early treatment of congenital hypothyroidism. *Pediatrics* **84:** 785–788.

Foley TP, Malvaux P & Blizzard RM (1994) Thyroid disease. In Kappy MS, Blizzard RM & Migeon CJ (eds) *The Diagnosis and Treatment of Endocrine Disorders in Childhood and Adolescence,* pp 457–533. Springfield, IL: Charles Thomas.

Fuggle PW, Grant DB, Smith I & Murphy G (1991) Intelligence, motor skills and behaviour at 5 years in early treated congenital hypothyroidism. *European Journal of Pediatrics* **159:** 570–574.

Glorieux J, Dussault JH, Morrisette J et al (1985) Follow up at ages 5 and 7 years on mental development in children with congenital hypothyroidism checked by the screening programme. *Journal of Pediatrics* **107:** 913–915.

Glorieux J, Dussault JH & Van Vliet G (1992) Intellectual development at 12 years in children with congenital hypothyroidism diagnosed by neonatal screening. *Journal of Pediatrics* **121:** 581–584.

Glorieux J, Desjardins M, Letarte J et al (1988) Useful parameters to predict the eventual mental outcome of hypothyroid children. *Pediatric Research* **24:** 6–8.

Grüters A, Delange F & Giovannelli G (1993) Guidelines for neonatal screening programmes for congenital hypothyroidism. *European Journal of Pediatrics* **152:** 974–975.

Grüters A, Liesenkötter KP & Willgerodt H (1995) Persistence of difference in iodine status in newborns after the reunification in Berlin. *New England Journal of Medicine* **333:** 1429.

Grüters A, l'Allemand D, Heidemann P & Schürnbrand P (1983) Incidence of iodine contamination in neonatal transient hyperthyreotropinemia. *European Journal of Pediatrics* **140:** 299–301.

Grüters A, Finke R, Krude H & Meinhold H (1994) Etiological grouping of permanent congenital hypothyroidism with a gland in situ. *Hormone Research* **41:** 3–9.

Harada S, Ichihara N, Arai J et al (1995) Later manifestations of congenital hypothyroidism predicted by slightly elevated thyrotropin levels in neonatal screening. *Screening* **3:** 181–192.

Heyerdahl S, Kase BF & Lie SO (1991) Intellectual development in children with congenital hypothyroidism in relation to recommended thyroxine treatment. *Journal of Pediatrics* **118:** 850–857.

Illicki A & Larsson A (1991) Psychological development at 7 years of age in children with congenital hypothyroidism. *Acta Paediatrica Scandinavica* **80:** 199–204.

Illig R & Rodiguez de vera R (1976) Radioimmunologischer Nachweis von TSH in getrockneten Blutstropfen: mögliche Screeningmethode zur Entdeckung der angeborenen Hypothyreose. *Schweizer Medizinische Wochenschrift* **106:** 1676–1681.

Illig R, Largo RH, Torresani T et al (1987) Mental development in congenital hypothyroidism after neonatal screening. *Archives of Disease in Childhood* **62:** 1050–1055.

Klein AH, Meltzer S & Kenny FH (1972) Improved prognosis in congenital hypothyroidism treated before age three months. *Journal of Pediatrics* **81:** 912–916.

Kooistra L, Laane C, Vulsma T et al (1994) Motor and cognitive development in children with congenital hypothyroidism: a long-term evaluation of the effects of neonatal treatment. *Journal of Pediatrics* **124:** 903–909.

l'Allemand D, Grüters A, Beyer P & Weber B (1987) Iodine in contrast agents and skin disinfectants is the major cause of hypothyroidism in premature infants during intensive care. *Hormone Research* **28:** 42–48.

Letarte J, Dussault JH, Guyda H et al (1981) Clinical and laboratory investigations in hypothyroid infants. In Collu R (ed.) *Pediatric Endocrinology*, pp 433–440. New York: Raven Press.

Matsuura N, Yamada Y & Nohara Y (1980) Familial transient hypothyroidism due to maternal TSH binding inhibitory immunoglobulins. *New England Journal of Medicine* **303:** 738–741.

Mitchell ML, Hermos RJ, Frederick DL & Klein RZ (1989) Problems in the management of patients with infantile hypothyroidism. In Delange F, Fischer DA & Glinoer D (eds) *Research in Congenital Hypothyroidism*, pp 237–244. New York: Plenum Press.

New England Congenital Hypothyroidism Collaborative (1990) Elementary school performance of children with congenital hypothyroidism. *Journal of Pediatrics* **116:** 27–32.

New England Congenital Hypothyroidism Collaborative (1985) Neonatal hypothyroidism screening: status of patients at 6 years of age. *Journal of Pediatrics* **107:** 915–918.

Pipanon C, Santos A & Perez-Castillo A (1992) Thyroid hormone up-regulates NGFI-A gene expression in rat brain during development. *Journal of Biological Chemistry* **267:** 21–23.

Refetoff S, Weiss RE & Usala SK (1993) The syndromes of resistance to thyroid hormone. *Endocrine Reviews* **14:** 348–399.

Rezvani I & DiGeorge AM (1977) Reassessment of the daily dose thyroxine for replacement therapy in hypothyroid children. *Journal of Pediatrics* **90:** 291–295.

Rochiccioli P, Dutau G, Despert F et al (1984) La surface des epiphses de genou index d'anciennete de l'hypothyroidie neonatale. *Archives Francaises de Pediatrie* **41:** 329–332.

Rovet JF (1992) Neurodevelopmental outcome in infants and preschool children following newborn screening for congenital hypothyroidism. *Journal of Pediatric Psychology* **17:** 187–213.

Rovet J & Ehrlich RM (1995) Longterm effects of l-thyroxine treatment for congenital hypothyroidism. *Journal of Pediatrics* **126:** 380–386.

Rovet J, Ehrlich R & Sorbara D (1987) Intellectual outcome in children with fetal hypothyroidism. *Journal of Pediatrics* **110:** 700–704.

Simons WF, Fuggle PW, Grand DB & Smith I (1994) Intellectual development at 10 years in early treated congenital hypothyroidism. *Archives of Disease in Childhood* **71:** 232–234.

Stein A, Shanklin DR, Adams PM et al (1989) Thyroid hormone regulation of specific mRNAs in the developing brain. In Delong GR, Robbins J & Condliffe PG (eds) *Iodine*, pp 59–78. New York: Plenum Press.

Tillotson SL, Fuggle PW, Smith I et al (1994) Relation between biochemical severity and intelligence in early treated congenital hypothyroidism: a threshold effect. *British Medical Journal* **309:** 440–445.

Toublanc JE, & the ESPE Working Group on Congenital Hypothyroidism (1990a) Epidemiological inquiry on congenital hypothyroidism in Europe. *Hormone Research* **34:** 1–3.

Toublanc JE, & the ESPE Working Group on Congenital Hypothyroidism (1992) Comparison of epidemiological data on congenital hypothyroidism in Europe with those of other parts in the world. *Hormone Research* **38:** 230–235.

Toublanc JE, Rives S, Ascota A & Chicaud J (1990b) Le development psychomoteur et intellectuel chez 52 enfants atteints d'hypotyroidie congenitale depistée a la naissance. *Archives Francais Pediatrie* **47:** 191–195.

van der Gaag RD, Drexhage H & Dussault J (1985) Role of maternal immunoglobulins blocking TSH induced thyroid growth in the sporadic forms of congenital hypothyroidism. *Lancet* **ii:** 246–250.

Virtanen M, Santavouri P, Hirvonen E & Peerheentupa J (1989) Multivariate analysis of psychomotor development in congenital hypothyroidism. *Acta Paediatrica Scandinavica* **78:** 405–411.

Vulsma T, Gons M & de Vijlder JJM (1989) Maternal–fetal transfer of thyroxine in congenital hypothyroidism due to a total organification defect or thyroid dysgenesis. *New England Journal of Medicine* **321:** 13–16.

Walfish PG, Ginsberg J, Rosenberg RA & Howard NJ (1979) Results of a regional cord blood screening program for detection of congenital hypothyroidism. *Archives of Diseases in Childhood* **54:** 171.

Zegher F de & Vanderschueren-Lodewyckx M (1989) Congenital hypothyroidism and monoamniotic twins. *Lancet* **ii:** 169–170.

4

Optimizing the management of congenital adrenal hyperplasia

TIM D. CHEETHAM
IEUAN A. HUGHES

The adrenal cortex converts cholesterol by a series of enzymatic steps to one of three principle steroid products: cortisol, aldosterone and androgens. Congenital adrenal hyperplasia (CAH) is the term used to describe a group of autosomal recessive disorders where the activity of one of the enzymes responsible for normal adrenal steroid production is reduced or absent. With a knowledge of the adrenal steroid pathway and the properties of the various steroid intermediates, some of the consequences of a given enzyme defect can usually be determined. In the most common form of CAH, 21-hydroxylase (21-OH) deficiency, the normal pathway to cortisol and aldosterone is affected so that operation of the classic negative feedback loop leads to the enhanced production of adrenal sex steroids. 21-OH deficiency is the underlying enzyme defect in approximately 95% of cases of CAH and is therefore considered in greatest detail in this review.

CAH carries with it a well-recognized morbidity. Complications of the disorder include inappropriate sex assignment, adrenal 'crises' at times of intercurrent illness, continuing virilization of affected females, impaired fertility and a reduced final adult height. The management of children and adolescents with established CAH due to 21-OH deficiency aims to ensure normal or near-normal growth and development by preventing the complications of androgen excess and glucocorticoid deficiency. Beyond puberty, it is to be hoped that levels of well-being, sexuality and fertility are no different from those of unaffected individuals.

This chapter highlights some of the more recent advances in the understanding of CAH that are relevant to the clinician. These include discussion of the genetics, prenatal diagnosis and treatment, neonatal screening, biochemical monitoring and therapy of CAH, which have all received particular attention over the past decade.

THE ADRENAL CORTEX

The adrenal cortex consists of two principle layers in the fetus and young infant—the inner fetal zone and outer adult zone. At this stage, the adult or

Baillière's Clinical Paediatrics—
Vol. 4, No. 2, May 1996
ISBN 0–7020–2180–6
0963–6714/96/020277 + 17 $12.00/00

definitive layer can also be subdivided into two zones—the outer glomerulosa and inner fasciculata. Adrenal and placental steroidogenesis are closely linked in utero; the enzyme activities are complementary, and together they play a major role as regulators of oestrogen production from steroid precursors. In infancy, the fetal zone involutes, and then in later childhood the adult zone acquires a third layer with the appearance of the zona reticularis. The three layers, which together comprise the mature adrenal cortex, demonstrate a degree of functional as well as anatomical independence, the glomerulosa producing mineralocorticoids, the fasciculata, glucocorticoids, and the reticularis, androgens. The development of the zona reticularis is associated with the appearance of the clinical signs of androgen action at adrenarche observed in some normal children at around 7 years of age. The adrenal androgens (androstenedione, dihydro-epiandrosterone [DHA] and its sulphate) are produced in increasing amounts during puberty, to reach maximum concentrations in late adolescence. These steroids are relatively weak androgens but can be converted peripherally to more potent androgens, such as testosterone. The adrenal biosynthetic pathway is shown in Figure 1.

ACTH is the principle trophic factor determining cortisol release, while aldosterone secretion is controlled primarily by the renin–angiotensin system and by serum electrolyte concentrations (particularly serum potassium levels). The relative morphological and functional indepen-dence of the zonae fasciculata and glomerulosa is also apparent from clinical studies of 11β-hydroxylase (11β-OH) deficiency (Spoudeas et al, 1993), although adrenocorticotrophic hormone (ACTH) does affect mineralocorticoid homeostasis, which is an important consideration when monitoring treatment in CAH. Adrenal androgen levels in patients with ACTH resistance (characterized by low cortisol but markedly elevated ACTH concentrations) are also reduced, which illustrates that ACTH is an important regulator of zona reticularis activity as well (Weber et al, 1995).

NORMAL ADRENAL STEROID PRODUCTION

ACTH and cortisol are released in a pulsatile manner in infancy, child-hood and adolescence (Wallace et al, 1991; Kerrigan et al, 1993; Metzger et al, 1993; de Zegher et al, 1994). Total plasma cortisol concentrations fall on the first day of life, and morning levels (08.00–10.00 h) then rise steadily during childhood and adolescence (Rokicki et al, 1990; Jonetz-Mentzel and Wiedemann, 1993). The normal circadian rhythm can be identified by 3–9 months of age (Price et al, 1983; Kiess et al, 1995). Beyond infancy, adrenal androgen production is low until the develop-ment of the zona reticularis just prior to puberty. There is no clear circadian rhythm to androgen release by the adrenal cortex. Mineralo-corticoid is produced at a relatively constant rate throughout childhood and adolescence.

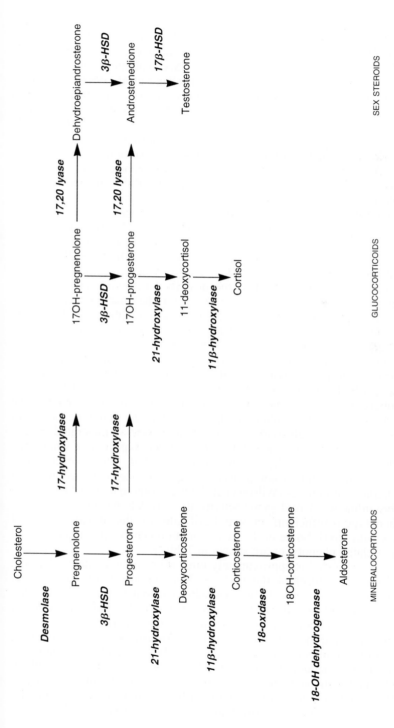

Figure 1. Pathways of adrenal steroidogenesis. 3β-HSD = 3β-hydroxysteroid dehydrogenase; 17β-HSD = 17β-hydroxysteroid dehydrogenase.

INCIDENCE AND GENETICS OF CAH

The incidence of CAH due to 21-OH deficiency is around 1 in 10 000–17 000 in Western Europe and the USA, with an overall worldwide figure of approximately 1 in 14 000 births (Pang et al, 1988). The Yupik eskimos of Alaska have a particularly high incidence, with figures of 1 in 490 derived from case ascertainment but 1 in 280 by screening programmes.
There are two 21-OH genes, one of which is the active *CYP21B* gene and the other the inactive *CYP21A* gene. They are located on the short arm of chromosome 6 in the midst of the major histocompatibility complex (HLA complex) and interspersed between the two genes encoding for the C4 components of complement. 21-OH is a cytochrome P450 enzyme bound to endoplasmic reticulum, where it is responsible for converting progesterone to deoxycorticosterone, and 17-hydroxyprogesterone (17-OHP) to 11-deoxycortisol. Most individuals with CAH due to 21-OH deficiency are compound heterozygotes. The majority of *CYP21* gene mutations are micro or macro conversions, in which part of the active 21-OH gene (*P450c21B*) is converted to the inactive gene (*P450c21A*), or where a section of the gene is deleted. Interestingly, most of the described deletions have not been random but occur from a specific point on the inactive gene to the corresponding point on the active gene, thereby creating a hybrid gene composed of inactive and active gene segments. Table 1 summarizes the more frequent mutations that have been identified. Most individuals with the severe salt-wasting form of CAH have gene deletions or conversions that severely impair enzyme activity, in contrast to mild, non-classical disease in which gene disruption is less marked (Speiser et al, 1992). Thus individuals with large gene conversions and gene deletions tend to be classical salt-wasters (Collier et al, 1989). *CYP21* genotype does not always correlate closely with phenotype, however, as illustrated by the report of two siblings with an identical *CYP21* genotype, one of whom was a salt-loser whereas the other was not (Bormann et al, 1992). Noncordance between genotype and phenotype has subsequently been demonstrated in a larger number of families (Wilson et al, 1995a). Although other factors may therefore influence steroidogenic activity, the correlation between genotype and phenotype is sufficiently close to be of value in clinical management of families with CAH. Some of the more common genetic abnormalities and their associated phenotypes are shown in Table 1.
Salt-wasting CAH is approximately three times more common than the simple virilizing form of the disease (Pang et al, 1988). The factors determining sodium status have been subject to much discussion, but the analysis of mutant enzymes re-created in vitro indicates that it is a function of the relative amount of gene product (mineralocorticoid and glucocorticoid) required to maintain homeostasis. Aldosterone levels equivalent to 0.1% of those of cortisol will maintain steady state, and, in the presence of reduced enzyme activity, affected individuals are therefore more likely to have glucocorticoid deficiency alone, and hence be simple virilizers. Competitive inhibition of mineralocorticoid action in vivo by the markedly elevated concentration of intermediates in CAH (such as 17-OHP) and the

Table 1. The relationship between mutation, allele frequency and phenotype in CAH.

Mutation (CYP 21)	Allele frequency (%)	Clinical state
Gene deletion (resulting in A/B 'hybrid')	15	SW
Gene macroconversions (Part of 'B' converted to 'A')	10	SW
A–G Intron 2 (resulting in more than one RNA splice variant)	20–25	SW (usually)
Microconversions		
Ile 172→Asn	20	SV
Val 281→Leu	6	NC
8 bp deletion	3–5	SW
Arg 356→Trp	3	SV
Pro 30→Leu	2	NC

SW = salt-wasting; SV = simple virilizing; NC = non-classical.

relatively immature renal tubular function in the neonatal period are also factors that influence sodium balance.

CLINICAL PRESENTATION OF CAH

CAH classically presents as ambiguous genitalia in an affected female, and 21-OH deficiency is the most common cause of intersex in the newborn. The diagnosis is virtually established in the presence of a 46XX karyotype and no palpable gonads. Female patients typically have an enlarged clitoris and varying degrees of labioscrotal fold fusion, which, at the more severe end of the spectrum, may lead to incorrect sex assignment because of a prominent phallus and a phallic urethra. The internal female organs develop normally because Müllerian inhibiting hormone (produced by the testes) is absent. Male infants may have genital hyperpigmentation but are not excessively virilized, and an underlying error of steroidogenesis is not usually suspected at birth. Most of these infants will subsequently present with a salt-losing crisis in the first weeks of life or, in the case of simple virilizing CAH, later in childhood with a clinical picture of pseudoprecocious puberty in which there are signs of pubertal development but no testicular enlargement. Female patients who are not identified at birth may also present with pseudoprecocious puberty or with signs suggestive of an early or pronounced adrenarche. Appropriate investigations in a child with ambiguous genitalia are listed in Table 2. Pelvic ultrasonography is a useful means of demonstrating a normal uterus and ovaries in an affected female. Enlarged adrenals with what has been described as a characteristic 'cerebriform' appearance may be visualized at the same time (Avni et al, 1993). A urinary steroid profile determined by gas chromatography and mass spectrometry is a valuable investigative tool and is considered by many to be of fundamental importance (Honour and Rumsby, 1993). A sample of urine (at least 10 ml) should always be saved for analysis at a later date in case there is difficulty reaching a diagnosis. Case reports of children with adrenal tumours but biochemical results suggestive of CAH serve to emphasize the importance of comprehensive assessment (Werder et al, 1994).

Table 2. Appropriate investigations in a case of suspected CAH and useful parameters when monitoring progress on treatment.

Investigations	Monitoring treatment
Karyotype	Growth
17-OHP	17-OHP
Testosterone	Testosterone
11-deoxycortisol	Electrolytes
Electrolytes (Na⁺, K⁺, urea, creatinine)	Plasma renin activity
Blood glucose	(Salivary/blood spot steroid profiles if available)
Urinary electrolytes	
Plasma renin activity	
Pelvic and renal ultrasound	

When investigating mineralocorticoid status in a neonate, the first indication may be a rising serum potassium and low serum sodium level (Brook, 1990). Urinary electrolytes may also be a useful guide during this initial phase, and mineralocorticoid deficiency would be suspected in the presence of a low-to-normal serum sodium but a relatively high urinary sodium output. Determining plasma renin activity may also be useful, although the delay between sampling and obtaining a result limits the value of this investigation in the neonatal period. It is also worth noting that plasma renin activity is normally elevated in healthy neonates compared with older children, so appropriate reference values need to be used.

SALT-LOSING CRISES

Approximately 75% of patients with CAH due to 21-OH deficiency have a relative deficiency of mineralocorticoid, and when a salt-losing tendency cannot be overcome by compensatory mechanisms, the classical clinical picture of a salt-losing crisis occurs. This is usually within the first 6 weeks of life; in a recent study (Donaldson et al, 1994), the age of presentation ranged from 5 to 42 days (median 12). In Sweden between 1969 and 1986, the median age at diagnosis of salt-losing boys was 21 days (Thilén and Larsson, 1990). Such infants typically present with a history of poor weight gain, vomiting and signs of hypovolaemia and a characteristic electrolyte imbalance (hyponatraemia, hyperkalaemia and an elevated urea level). Glucocorticoid deficiency may also manifest as hypoglycaemia. Such adrenal crises usually occur in affected males who lack the genital signs which facilitate earlier diagnosis in the affected female. However, severely virilized females may also present acutely with mineralocorticoid deficiency. There is usually little doubt as to the underlying diagnosis once the child has been assessed and the biochemical results are available. Nevertheless, an obstructed renal tract may present similar findings; this is a potential source of some confusion, so a renal ultrasound early in the course of the illness is a useful investigation. Treatment of affected CAH infants centres on the correction of hypoglycaemia and volume replacement with fluids of a high sodium content and glucocorticoids.

MANAGEMENT

The final height of adults with CAH is usually compromised. Perhaps this is an inevitable consequence of the disease, but more appropriate treatment and improvements in management should reduce the impact of the disorder on stature. Glucocorticoids and sex steroids both have profound effects on growth. The growth-suppressive effects of glucocorticoids are well established. Excess androgens in pre-puberty increase the growth rate and rapidly advance bone maturation, so that final height is compromised because of a curtailment of the normal period of pre-pubertal growth. There are numerous reports of over-treatment with signs of glucocorticoid excess, and under-treatment with subsequent rapid growth, advanced bone age and a similar deleterious impact on final height.

The aim of glucocorticoid replacement in CAH is to suppress excess androgen production with the minimum dose that also allows growth to occur at a normal rate. The balance between rate of growth and skeletal maturation is of fundamental importance when monitoring the treatment of CAH. Whether it is practical in CAH to attain a normal rate of growth in the presence of normal plasma steroid concentrations for age is not known. It has been suggested that the intrinsic defect in adrenal steroidogenesis will still lead to excess androgens when replacement doses of glucocorticoid and mineralocorticoid are used, and ACTH production is normalized (Young et al, 1989). Recent studies indicate that the normal endogenous cortisol production rate is less than that calculated previously. Values of around 6–7 mg/m^2 per day have been derived from studies undertaken in childhood and adolescence, using separate and reliable methodologies (Linder et al, 1990; Kerrigan et al, 1993). Given a bioavailability of orally administered hydrocortisone of around 50% (although this can vary considerably from 26–91%), a replacement dose of hydrocortisone is therefore likely to be in the region of 12–15 mg/m^2 per day. The dose required to suppress androgen levels may be greater than this (20–25 mg/m^2 per day), which may reflect the extent of the enzyme deficiency as well as differences in glucocorticoid bioavailability (Sandrini et al, 1993). Consequently, the use of anti-androgen drugs such as flutamide, and aromatase inhibitors such as testolactone, in combination with glucocorticoid replacement has been proposed as a novel alternative treatment regimen (Cutler and Laue, 1990). By this means, physiological doses of glucocorticoid might be used without the deleterious impact of excess androgen on final height.

Hydrocortisone is commonly administered in childhood and can safely be given twice or three times daily even though the half-life is only 90 minutes. Hydrocortisone is rapidly absorbed, and the largest dose is usually given in the morning to mimic the normal diurnal pattern of cortisol secretion. Replacement doses of hydrocortisone may be used to treat infants from the outset (Young and Hughes, 1990), and it appears that frequent adjustment of the dose in the first year of life is probably unnecessary (Thilén et al, 1995). It is an intriguing observation that although androgen levels in male CAH infants are elevated at birth and in the initial months of life, the genitalia appear to be relatively unresponsive at this stage. Beyond the first year of life, children should be reviewed at 3–6

monthly intervals, depending on current growth rate and the results of biochemical investigations. Adolescent and adult patients are often managed
with once daily dexamethasone, and there is evidence to suggest that this is
not only more straightforward, but that ovarian function in females may
also be improved (Horrocks and London, 1987). Dexamethasone is not
always well tolerated, and both the dose and steroid preparation used may
need to be tailored to the individual (Horrocks and London, 1987).

Most young infants with mineralocorticoid deficiency require oral sodium
supplements (approximately 2 mmol/kg per day initially) in addition to
mineralocorticoid. These can usually be withdrawn once weaning is established. In older children, a relative lack of mineralocorticoid may not be
manifest as altered serum electrolytes, and a salt-losing tendency needs to be
considered in all children with CAH. Mineralocorticoid activity is
influenced by the hypothalamo–pituitary–adrenal axis as well as the
renin–angiotensin system, so inadequate aldosterone production may lead to
increased ACTH-induced androgen synthesis despite apparently sufficient
glucocorticoid replacement (Hughes et al, 1979). Salt loss may therefore be
manifest as difficulty in achieving adequate control on glucocorticoid
replacement alone, and can be identified by the measurement of plasma
renin activity as a more sensitive index of mineralocorticoid replacement.
The dose of mineralocorticoid is usually around 100–150 $\mu g/m^2$ per 24
hours in older children, although larger amounts may be required in infancy.

Surgical management of CAH

Correction of the virilized external genitalia in affected females is usually
a two-stage procedure, involving a reduction in clitoral size and a later
reconstruction of the vagina. The complexity of both procedures is clearly
linked to the degree of virilization; this is a major undertaking when the
vagina is located above the level of the external urethral sphincter (Hendren
and Atala, 1995). Surgery at a later stage may still be needed to help ensure
an adequate vaginal outlet (Bailez et al, 1992). Early assessment by an
experienced paediatric urologist is an important part of the management of
any virilized female.

INTERCURRENT ILLNESS AND SURGERY

Guidelines regarding the management of intercurrent illness should be
discussed with the family prior to discharge from hospital following
diagnosis. The dose of glucocorticoid should be trebled at the time of stress,
such as a significant febrile illness or episodes of diarrhoea or vomiting.
There is evidence from studies in normal children that a more aggressive
increase may be appropriate in severe illness (Levine et al, 1994). The
family also need to be instructed in the use of an injectable form of glucocorticoid, such as hydrocortisone phosphate, to cover severe illness when
the child becomes unwell quickly, or when vomiting prevents oral glucocorticoid administration. There is evidence that such measures reduce

morbidity (Donaldson et al, 1994). There is no need to alter the dose of mineralocorticoid at the time of such illnesses.

The dose of glucocorticoid requires adjustment at the time of routine or emergency surgery. It has been estimated that the endogenous production of cortisol doubles at such times of 'stress'. The extra or increased dose of glucocorticoid is usually administered at induction at the time of routine surgery and can usually be reduced to pre-surgical levels in the subsequent 48 hours. Ongoing sepsis or the development of other complications necessitates continued treatment at increased levels.

MONITORING TREATMENT

A combination of auxological and biochemical parameters is commonly used to monitor treatment in CAH, although detailed clinical assessment is also important (Sane and Pescovitz, 1992). An appropriate height velocity in the absence of androgen excess is the desired end-point, and biochemical indices can be a useful adjunct to achieving this objective. Plasma or salivary steroid levels (17-OHP, testosterone and androstenedione) can be determined at specific times or as a 'profile' throughout the day. The results are interpreted in relation to the timing of treatment and compared with normal steroid rhythms. Steroid profiles have become easier to perform now that samples can be collected as blood spots on filter paper; they are a useful index of control, and nomograms have been developed which help to interpret the results (Young et al, 1988a, b). Salivary 17-OHP concentrations can also be assessed, although this is usually limited to older children who are able to provide the required samples. A correlation between 17-OHP profiles and growth rate has been identified, and an average height velocity appears to be related to suppression of 17-OHP concentrations but maintainance of a significant diurnal variation. An abnormally rapid rate of growth and bone maturation is associated with non-suppressed plasma or blood spot 17-OHP (>40 nmol/l), whereas steroid over-replacement, as identified by significantly decreased height velocity, is associated with suppression of plasma/blood spot 17-OHP concentrations to below 10 nmol/l throughout the day (Pincus et al, 1993). Measurement of urinary 17-OHP excretion is also currently being assessed as a monitor of control (Lim et al, 1995). Plasma renin activity, ideally measured in the morning, is a valuable index of mineralocorticoid activity and thus a guide to the adequacy of salt balance.

NEONATAL SCREENING

The diagnosis in most infants and children with CAH is made relatively promptly and reflects the increased awareness of the condition by medical and nursing staff. If all affected individuals were identified, the expected male to female ratio in CAH would be 1:1. A female preponderance of CAH was identified in the West Midlands (UK) before 1970 (Virdi et al,

1987) and in Wales between 1966 and 1977 (Murtaza et al, 1980). More recently, the ratio has approached the expected figure (Virdi et al, 1987). Deaths from undiagnosed CAH still occur, and the development of assays that can measure 17-OHP levels on blood spot samples collected at the time of routine screening for other conditions (hypothyroidism and phenylketonuria, for example) has focused attention on the early identification of CAH. The principal argument for screening newborn infants with 21-OH deficiency is to prevent a salt-losing crisis or hypoglycaemia in male infants. Affected females should be ascertained by careful newborn examination, although the occasional infant with isolated and mild clitoromegaly has been missed. The case for screening can be extended to include the prevention of androgen excess and later problems associated with growth. An effective neonatal screening programme should identify affected infants rapidly—in practice within 10 days of birth—and not be influenced by excessive numbers of false positive results. Spuriously elevated concentrations of 17-OHP can occur in sick infants, especially those who are preterm. Even though a pilot screening programme in Scotland showed promising results (Wallace et al, 1986), it was decided not to add CAH to the UK national screening programmes that use the newborn Guthrie cards. In the USA, the screening programme is an integral part of newborn care in a number of states (Pang et al, 1988), as it is in other countries, such as New Zealand (Cutfield and Webster, 1995).

PRENATAL DIAGNOSIS AND TREATMENT

The prenatal diagnosis of CAH was initially based on the measurement of steroid precursors in amniotic fluid (Jeffcoate et al, 1965; Hughes et al, 1987), and the prenatal treatment of two affected pregnancies was subsequently described (David and Forest, 1984). Virilization of affected females occurs early in fetal life; available evidence now suggests that prenatal treatment of CAH with steroids has a beneficial effect on the degree of masculinization of female infants when begun in early pregnancy, but this remains an experimental procedure (Miller, 1994).

A plan outlining the approach to the prenatal diagnosis and treatment of CAH is illustrated in Figure 2. It is important to establish the 21-OH genotype of the index case and relevant family members in advance of planning a further pregnancy. Amniocentesis and chorionic villus sampling are not without risk to the fetus—the incidence of miscarriage is around 0.3 and 0.8% respectively—and this clearly needs to be considered at the outset. Congenital malformations have also been linked to chorionic villus sampling and need to be discussed. The mother should begin glucocorticoid treatment once pregnancy has been confirmed (ideally by 6 weeks gestation). Treatment is usually administered in the form of a synthetic steroid such as dexamethasone (20 µg/kg per day in 2–3 divided doses) and is intended to suppress fetal and maternal adrenal function. Dexamethasone is generally used because it is not inactivated by placental 11β-hydroxysteroid dehydrogenase to the same extent as are other glucocorticoids. The

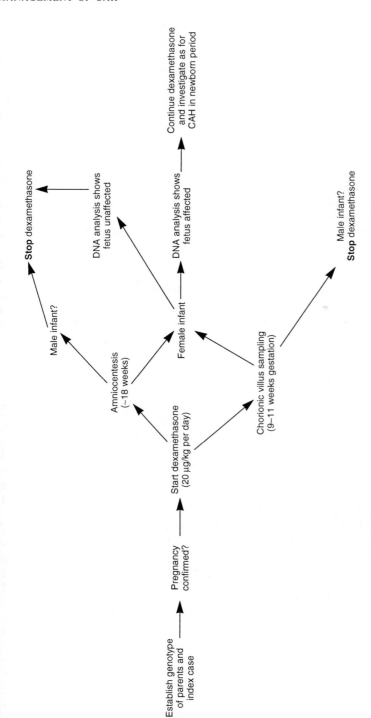

Figure 2. Flow diagram outlining an approach to the prenatal diagnosis and treatment of CAH.

karyotype of the fetus can be identified at the earliest opportunity and DNA obtained, either by chorionic villus sampling at 9–11 weeks or by amniocentesis at 15–18 weeks. Genetic analysis of fetal DNA and comparison with the genotype of the index case and the parents will indicate in which pregnancies steroid treatment needs to be continued; it can be stopped if the fetus is male and (on average) in the three out of four females who do not have the same 21-OH genotype as the affected sibling. If the fetus is female and has a genotype compatible with CAH, treatment is continued throughout pregnancy.

DNA analysis was initially undertaken by linkage studies that made use of the proximity of the 21-OH gene to the HLA locus, whereas specific DNA probes can now be used to screen for known mutations (Speiser et al, 1994). With a knowledge of the genotype of parents and affected siblings, a structured approach to the analysis of the genotype of chorionic villus samples can be used, so that treatment of unaffected pregnancies may be terminated at an earlier stage than if amniocentesis and HLA haplotyping are used for diagnosis. Diagnostic accuracy is generally high, but there can be problems, such as poor hybridization of the DNA probe or contamination of fetal with maternal cells (false negatives) and errors in interpretation (false positives). The use of allele-specific polymerase chain reaction and the increasing refinement of other molecular biological techniques will improve the speed and accuracy of genotype determination (Wilson et al, 1995b).

There are now reports of female CAH infants with normal female genitalia, in contrast to the era before prenatal intervention, although surgical intervention to improve the appearance and function of the genitalia may still be needed (Odink et al, 1988; Wudy et al, 1994). With early dexamethasone treatment, it was recently reported that of 7 affected female infants who had affected female siblings, 3 had normal female genitalia at birth, while the remainder had genitalia that were significantly less virilized than would otherwise have been expected (Mercado et al, 1995). There is also evidence of a reduction in virilization even when glucocorticoid treatment is delayed, so treatment of more mature pregnancies may be of some benefit.

The complications of steroid treatment in the mother include excessive weight gain, Cushingoid features, striae, glucose intolerance, increased blood pressure, mood fluctuations and gastrointestinal upset (Pang et al, 1992). There are no reported postnatal complications of prenatal treatment (affected or unaffected individuals), although follow-up data are limited (Forest et al, 1993). Careful monitoring of mother and fetus throughout pregnancy is clearly essential.

NON-CLASSICAL CAH

It is increasingly recognized that subtle reductions of 21-OH activity can present in a variety of ways in later childhood, adolescence and adult life. In childhood, this may manifest as virilization, which can potentially be confused with conditions such as premature adrenarche and virilizing adrenal tumours. 17-OHP secretion is enhanced in non-classical CAH, and mild abnormalities of cortisol release can also be identified (Ghizzoni et al, 1994). In later life, affected individuals may present with acne, menstrual irregularity and hirsutism. Where there is concern about non-classical CAH, basal (ideally morning) 17-OHP concentrations, perhaps combined with ACTH stimulation testing, may help to distinguish between normal and abnormal adrenal steroid production (Balducci et al, 1994). Nomograms have been published which can aid with the interpretation of androgen concentrations pre- and post-ACTH stimulation (Lashansky et al, 1991), although reference values will differ between laboratories, which should be borne in mind (Wallace, 1995).

OTHER CAUSES OF CAH

Other causes of CAH besides 21-OH deficiency need to be considered at the time of presentation. The most common is 11β-OH deficiency, which accounts for approximately 5–8% of cases but is more common in certain racial groups. Affected female infants typically present with marked signs of virilization, but there may also be evidence of salt and water retention, which classically leads to an elevated blood pressure beyond infancy. The affected enzyme in 11β-OH deficiency controls the final step in cortisol synthesis, so plasma 17-OHP levels, in addition to those of deoxycortisol, will be elevated (Figure 1). It is advisable to retain plasma routinely for deoxycortisol measurement in suspected CAH in case the criteria for 21-OH deficiency are not completely met. Hypertension in 11β-OH deficiency in later life is the result of the accumulation of potent mineralocorticoids such as deoxycorticosterone, but salt-wasting can also occur with this enzyme defect, especially when glucocorticoid replacement has been started (Zachmann et al, 1983).

The less common adrenal steroidogenic defects causing CAH require the measurement of urinary steroid excretion by specific chromatographic techniques.

MORBIDITY AND COMPLICATIONS

Numerous studies have shown the deleterious impact of CAH on growth and final adult height (Urban et al, 1978). Although genetic factors remain an important determinant of adult stature, the standard techniques for predicting final height must be interpreted with caution during childhood as they over-estimate adult height (Yu and Grant, 1995). In addition to the problems of salt-loss and virilization in childhood, poorly controlled CAH may lead to precocious puberty by premature activation of the hypo-thalamus–pituitary–gonadal axis, which will compromise growth still further. It remains to be established whether more detailed biochemical and auxological assessment during childhood will improve the outlook for growth.

Adrenal tumours have been described in children with untreated CAH and failure to reduce tumour size with glucocorticoid treatment has led to surgical removal (Bhatia et al, 1993). Benign tumours within the testes that have the morphological and enzymatic features suggestive of adrenal tissue (adrenal rests) are also described (Clark et al, 1990).

It has recently been shown that in a group of children with CAH, markers of bone turnover (osteocalcin and alkaline phosphatase) were reduced despite a normal growth rate (Lisa et al, 1995). This was thought to reflect continued androgen excess shown indirectly by elevated 17-OHP levels. The short- and long-term implications of the changes in bone metabolism are not known, but they serve to emphasize the link between endogenous steroid production and bone metabolism.

There is evidence in the longer term of an increased incidence of learning difficulties in CAH children, which has been linked to complications such as hypoglycaemia (Donaldson et al, 1994).

FERTILITY

Prospects for fertility are usually good in male patients with CAH (Urban et al, 1978), but affected individuals should remain on glucocorticoid treatment to prevent impaired gonadotrophin secretion and perhaps the development of testicular adrenal rest tumours. The fertility of affected females, in contrast, is relatively poor, with reported rates of 40% (Mulaikal et al, 1987). Decreased fertility is the result of a number of factors, including an inadequate vaginal introitus, poor compliance or inadequate treatment leading to menstrual cycle irregularity and anovulation.

The implications of exposure of the immature brain to excessive androgens has been of particular interest to researchers. Female patients with CAH may have decreased libido, fewer sexual encounters and an increased incidence of bisexual and homosexual fantasies (Mulaikal et al, 1987; Dittmann et al, 1992). A more masculine cognitive pattern has also been described (Helleday et al, 1994). To what extent these features are the result of prenatal androgen excess is not known, but the outcome of prenatal treatment on psychosexual development is clearly of major importance in the longer term.

SUMMARY

Significant advances in the molecular genetics and biochemical pathophysiology of CAH have occurred in recent years. However, a significant morbidity persists. Careful patient supervision and biochemical assessment may enhance final adult height, but the need for reconstructive surgery in most affected females persists. A greater understanding of the mechanism of action of sex steroids on growth, development and brain function should lead to improved treatment schedules for patients in future.

REFERENCES

Avni EF, Rypens F, Smet MH & Galetty E (1993) Sonographic demonstration of congenital adrenal hyperplasia in the neonate: the cerebriform pattern. *Pediatric Radiology* **23:** 88–90.

Bailez MM, Gearhart JP, Migeon C & Rock J (1992) Vaginal reconstruction after initial construction of the external genitalia in girls with salt-wasting adrenal hyperplasia. *Journal of Urology* **48:** 680–682.

Balducci R, Boscherini B, Mangiantini A et al (1994) Isolated precocious pubarche: an approach. *Journal of Clinical Endocrinology and Metabolism* **79:** 582–589.

Bhatia V, Shukla R, Mishra SK & Gupta RK (1993) Adrenal tumor complicating untreated 21-hydroxylase deficiency in a 5½-year-old boy. *American Journal of Diseases in Children* **147:** 1321–1323.

Bormann M, Kochhan L, Knorr D et al (1992) Clinical heterogeneity of 21-hydroxylase deficiency of sibs with identical 21-hydroxylase genes. *Acta Endocrinologica* **126:** 7–9.

Brook CGD (1990) The management of classical congenital adrenal hyperplasia due to 21-hydroxylase deficiency. *Clinical Endocrinology* **33:** 559–567.

Clark RV, Albertson BD, Munabi A et al (1990) Steroidogenic enzyme activities, morphology, and receptor studies of a testicular adrenal rest in a patient with congenital adrenal hyperplasia. *Journal of Clinical Endocrinology and Metabolism* **70:** 1408–1413.

Collier S, Sinnot PJ, Dyer PA et al (1989) Pulse field electrophoresis identifies a high degree of variability in the number of tandem 21-hydroxylase and complement C4 gene repeats in 21-hydroxylase haplotypes. *EMBO Journal* **8:** 1393–1402.

Cutfield WS & Webster D (1995) Newborn screening for congenital adrenal hyperplasia in New Zealand. *Journal of Pediatrics* **126:** 118–121.

Cutler GB & Laue L (1990) Congenital adrenal hyperplasia due to 21-hydroxylase deficiency. *New England Journal of Medicine* **323:** 1806–1813.

David M & Forest MG (1984) Prenatal treatment of congenital adrenal hyperplasia resulting from 21-hydroxylase deficiency. *Journal of Pediatrics* **105:** 799–803.

Dittmann RW, Kappes ME & Kappes MH (1992) Sexual behaviour in adolescent and adult females with congenital adrenal hyperplasia. *Psychoneuroendocrinology* **17:** 153–170.

Donaldson MDC, Thomas PH, Love JG et al (1994) Presentation, acute illness, and learning difficulties in salt-wasting 21-hydroxylase deficiency. *Archives of Disease in Childhood* **70:** 214–218.

Forest MG, David M & Morel Y (1993) Prenatal diagnosis and treatment of 21-hydroxylase deficiency. *Journal of Steroid Biochemistry and Molecular Biology* **45:** 75–82.

Ghizzoni L, Bernasconi S, Virdis R et al (1994) Dynamics of 24-hour pulsatile cortisol, 17-hydroxy-progesterone, and androstenedione release in prepubertal patients with nonclassic 21-hydroxylase deficiency and normal prepubertal children. *Metabolism* **43:** 372–377.

Helleday J, Bartfai A, Ritzen EM & Forsman M (1994) General intelligence and cognitive profile in women with congenital adrenal hyperplasia (CAH). *Psychoneuroendocrinology* **19:** 343–356.

Hendren WH & Atala A (1995) Repair of the high vagina in girls with severely masculinized anatomy from the adrenogenital syndrome. *Journal of Pediatric Surgery* **30:** 91–94.

Honour JW & Rumsby G (1993) Problems in diagnosis and management of congenital adrenal hyperplasia due to 21-hydroxylase deficiency. *Journal of Steroid Biochemistry and Molecular Biology* **45:** 69–74.

Horrocks PM & London DR (1987) Effects of long term dexamethasone treatment in adult patients with congenital adrenal hyperplasia. *Clinical Endocrinology* **27:** 635–642.

Hughes IA, Wilton A, Lole CA & Gray OP (1979) Continuing need for mineralocorticoid therapy in salt-losing congenital adrenal hyperplasia. *Archives of Disease in Childhood* **54:** 350–355.

Hughes IA, Dyas J, Riad-Fahmy D & Laurence KM (1987) Prenatal diagnosis of congenital adrenal hyperplasia: reliability of amniotic fluid steroid analysis. *Journal of Medical Genetics* **24:** 344–347.

Jeffcoate TNA, Fliegner JRH, Russel SH et al (1965) Diagnosis of the adrenogenital syndrome before birth. *Lancet* **ii:** 553–555.

Jonetz-Mentzel L & Wiedemann G (1993) Establishment of reference ranges for cortisol in neonates, infants, children and adolescents. *European Journal of Clinical Chemistry and Clinical Biochemistry* **31:** 525–529.

Kerrigan JR, Veldhuis JD, Leyo SA et al (1993) Estimation of daily cortisol production and clearance rates in normal pubertal males by deconvolution analysis. *Journal of Clinical Endocrinology and Metabolism* **76:** 1505–1510.

Kiess W, Meidert A, Dressendorfer RA et al (1995) Salivary cortisol levels throughout childhood and adolescence: relation with age, pubertal stage, and weight. *Pediatric Research* **37:** 502–506.

Lashansky G, Saenger P, Fishman K et al (1991) Normative data for adrenal steroidogenesis in a healthy pediatric population: age and sex-related changes after adrenocorticotropin stimulation. *Journal of Clinical Endocrinology and Metabolism* **73:** 674–686.

Levine A, Cohen D & Zadik Z (1994) Urinary free cortisol values in children under stress. *Journal of Pediatrics* **125:** 853–857.

Lim YJ, Yong AB, Warne GL & Montalto J (1995) Urinary 17-alpha-hydroxyprogesterone in management of 21-hydroxylase deficiency. *Journal of Paediatrics and Child Health* **31:** 47–50.

Linder BL, Esteban NV, Yergey AL et al (1990) Cortisol production rate in childhood and adolescence. *Journal of Pediatrics* **117:** 892–896.

Lisa L, Neradilova M, Tomasova N et al (1995) Osteocalcin in congenital adrenal hyperplasia. *Bone* **16:** 57–59.

Mercado AB, Wilson RC, Cheng KC et al (1995) Prenatal treatment and diagnosis of congenital adrenal hyperplasia owing to steroid 21-hydroxylase deficiency. *Journal of Clinical Endocrinology and Metabolism* **80:** 2014–2020.

Metzger DL, Wright NM, Veldhuis JD et al (1993) Characterization of pulsatile secretion and clearance of plasma cortisol in premature and term neonates using deconvolution analysis. *Journal of Clinical Endocrinology and Metabolism* **77:** 458–463.

Miller WL (1994) Genetics, diagnosis, and management of 21-hydroxylase deficiency. *Journal of Clinical Endocrinology and Metabolism* **78:** 241–246.

Mulaikal RM, Migeon CJ & Rock JA (1987) Fertility rates in patients with congenital adrenal hyperplasia due to 21-hydroxylase deficiency. *New England Journal of Medicine* **316:** 178–182.

Murtaza L, Sibert J, Hughes IA & Balfour IC (1980) Congenital adrenal hyperplasia—a clinical and genetic survey. Are we detecting male salt losers? *Archives of Disease in Childhood* **55:** 622–625.

Odink RJH, Boue A & Jansen M (1988) The value of chorion villus sampling in early detection of 21 hydroxylase deficiency (21-OHD). *Pediatric Research* **23:** 131A/156.

Pang S, Wallace AM, Hofman L et al (1988) Worldwide experience in newborn screening for classical congenital adrenal hyperplasia due to 21-hydroxylase deficiency. *Pediatrics* **81:** 866–874.

Pang S, Clark AT, Freeman LC et al (1992) Maternal side effects of prenatal dexamethasone therapy for fetal congenital adrenal hyperplasia. *Journal of Clinical Endocrinology and Metabolism* **75:** 249–253.

Pincus DR, Kelnar CJH & Wallace AM (1993) 17-hydroxyprogesterone rhythms and growth velocity in congenital adrenal hyperplasia. *Journal of Paediatrics and Child Health* **29:** 302–304.

Price DA, Close GC & Fielding BA (1983) Age of appearance of circadian rhythm in salivary cortisol values in normal children and adolescents. *Archives of Disease in Childhood* **58:** 454–456.

Rokicki W, Forest MG, Loras B et al (1990) Free cortisol of human plasma in the first three months of life. *Biology of the Neonate* **57:** 21–29.

Sandrini R, Jospe N & Migeon CJ (1993) Temporal and individual variations in the dose of gluco-corticoid used for the treatment of salt-losing congenital virilizing adrenal hyperplasia due to 21-hydroxylase deficiency. *Acta Paediatrica* **388 (supplement):** 56–60.

Sane K & Pescovitz OH (1992) The clitoral index: a determination of clitoral size in normal girls and in girls with abnormal sexual development. *Journal of Pediatrics* **120:** 264–266.

Speiser PW, Dupont J, Zhu D et al (1992) Disease expression and molecular genotype in congenital adrenal hyperplasia due to 21-hydroxylase deficiency. *Journal of Clinical Investigation* **90:** 584–595.

Speiser PW, White PC, Dupont J et al (1994) Prenatal diagnosis of congenital adrenal hyperplasia due to 21-hydroxylase deficiency by allele-specific hybridization and Southern blot. *Human Genetics* **93:** 424–428.

Spoudeas HA, Slater JDH, Rumsby G et al (1993) Deoxycorticosterone, 11β-hydroxylase and the adrenal cortex. *Clinical Endocrinology* **39:** 245–251.

Thilén A & Larsson A (1990) Congenital adrenal hyperplasia in Sweden 1969–1986. Prevalence, symptoms and age at diagnosis. *Acta Paediatrica* **79:** 168–175.

Thilén A, Woods KA, Perry LA et al (1995) Early growth is not increased in untreated moderately severe 21-hydroxylase deficiency. *Acta Paediatrica* **84:** 894–898.

Urban MD, Lee PA & Migeon CJ (1978) Adult height and fertility in men with congenital virilizing adrenal hyperplasia. *New England Journal of Medicine* **299:** 1392–1396.

Virdi NK, Rayner PHW, Rudd BT & Green A (1987) Should we screen for congenital adrenal hyperplasia? A review of 117 cases. *Archives of Disease in Childhood* **62:** 659–662.

Wallace AM (1995) Analytical support for the detection and treatment of congenital adrenal hyperplasia. *Annals of Clinical Biochemistry* **32:** 9–27.

Wallace AM, Beastall GH, Cook BA et al (1986) Neonatal screening for congenital adrenal hyperplasia: a programme based on a novel direct radioimmunoassay for 17-hydroxyprogesterone in blood spots. *Journal of Endocrinology* **108:** 299–308.

Wallace WHB, Crowne EC, Shalet SM et al (1991) Episodic ACTH and cortisol secretion in normal children. *Clinical Endocrinology* **34:** 215–221.

Weber A, Clark AJL, Shaw NJ et al (1995) Evidence for diminished adrenal androgen secretion with lack of adrenarche in patients with familial glucocorticoid deficiency. *Hormone Research* **44 (supplement 1):** 1A.

Werder EA, Voutilainen R & Zachmann M (1994) Virilizing adrenal tumour mimicking congenital adrenal hyperplasia with P450c11 (11β-hydroxylase) deficiency. *European Journal of Pediatrics* **153:** 411–415.

Wilson RC, Mercado AB, Cheng KC & New MI (1995a) Steroid 21-hydroxylase deficiency: genotype may not predict phenotype. *Journal of Clinical Endocrinology and Metabolism* **80:** 2322–2329.

Wilson RC, Wei J-Q, Cheng KC et al (1995b) Rapid deoxyribonucleic acid analysis by allele-specific polymerase chain reaction for detection of mutations in the steroid 21-hydroxylase gene. *Journal of Clinical Endocrinology and Metabolism* **80:** 1635–1640.

Wudy SA, Homoki J & Teller WM (1994) Successful prenatal treatment of congenital adrenal hyperplasia due to 21-hydroxylase deficiency. *European Journal of Pediatrics* **153:** 556–559.

Young MC & Hughes IA (1990) Response to treatment of congenital adrenal hyperplasia in infancy. *Archives of Disease in Childhood* **65:** 441–444.

Young MC, Ribeiro J & Hughes IA (1989) Growth and body proportions in congenital adrenal hyperplasia. *Archives of Disease in Childhood* **64:** 1554–1558.

Young MC, Robinson JA, Read GF et al (1988a) 170H-progesterone rhythms in congenital adrenal hyperplasia. *Archives of Disease in Childhood* **63:** 617–623.

Young MC, Walker RF, Riad-Fahmy D & Hughes IA (1988b) Androstenedione rhythms in saliva in congenital adrenal hyperplasia. *Archives of Disease in Childhood* **63:** 624–628.

Yu ACM & Grant DB (1995) Adult height in women with early-treated congenital adrenal hyperplasia (21-hydroxylase type): relation to body mass index in earlier childhood. *Acta Paediatrica* **84:** 899–903.

Zachmann M, Tassinari D & Prader A (1983) Clinical and biochemical variability of congenital adrenal hyperplasia due to 11β-hydroxylase deficiency. A study of 25 patients. *Journal of Clinical Endocrinology and Metabolism* **56:** 222–229.

Zegher FD de, Vanhole C, Van den Berghe G et al (1994) Properties of thyroid-stimulating hormone and cortisol secretion by the human newborn on the day of birth. *Journal of Clinical Endocrinology and Metabolism* **79:** 576–581.

5

Optimizing the management of Turner syndrome

MICHAEL B. RANKE

In 1938, Henry H. Turner described in seven females a disorder characterized by sexual infantilism, congenital webbed neck, cubitus valgus and
short stature. As early as 1930, Otto Ullrich had recognized the same disorder as a specific entity. Turner syndrome (TS) is caused by the absence
or structural abnormality of one X chromosome. Typical karyotypes are
45,X (approximately 50%), 46,X,i (Xq) and 46,X,rX. Normal and abnormal cell lines (e.g. 45,X/46,XX) may be combined (mosaicism). TS is a
rather frequent disorder (approximately 1 in 2500 liveborn phenotypical
females) that is characterized by three main clinical features (Ranke,

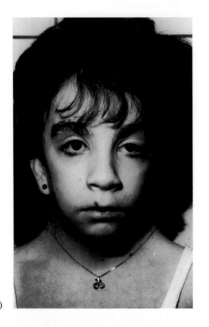 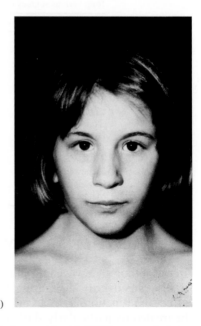

(a)   (b)

Figures 1(a) and (b). Variability of facial appearance in two girls with 45,X Turner syndrome.

Baillière's Clinical Paediatrics —
Vol. 4, No. 2, May 1996
ISBN 0–7020–2180–6
0963–6714/96/020295 + 13 $12.00/00

1989; Lippe, 1991): (a) abnormal external appearance and abnormalities of some internal organs, (b) malformation of the ovaries, and (c) short stature.

Deviation of the appearance (Figure 1) and abnormalities of internal organs varies. In some cases, the characteristic features allow the diagnosis *prima vista* and as early as in the neonatal phase (Table 1). In other cases, the features are subtle and need to be sought for. Gonadal dysgenesis progresses with age, thus allowing a fraction of patients to enter puberty (Hibi et al, 1991), and even allows fertility in rare cases. Short stature is the most constant finding in Turner syndrome. It is obvious that in such a complex situation, patient care must be equally complex. The problems related to different organ systems require specific medical expertise. However, TS is not just a combination of medical problems that may be more or less well corrected, but a disorder requiring a general concept of patient care that takes into consideration the long-term perspectives of the patient's life with all its medical and psychosocial aspects.

This review will focus on only a few important aspects among the multitude of different issues in comprehensive care. In a series of, so far, four international symposia (Rosenfeld and Grumbach, 1990; Ranke and Rosenfeld, 1991; Hibi and Takano, 1993; Albertsson-Wikland and Ranke, 1995) on Turner syndrome, many of the aspects were discussed in depth.

Table 1. Frequency of clinical abnormalities (%) collected from various sources in Turner syndrome ($N = 387$).

Symptoms/Area of symptoms	% of TS
Eyes	29
Ears	58
High arched palate	61
Neck/pterygium colli	67
Low-set hairline	80
Thorax	76
Cubitus valgus	50
Skin	72
Heart defect (all)	20
Pulmonary stenosis	Rare
Coarctation	14
Renal	57
Gonads	95
Mental retardation	11

TREATMENT OF ABNORMAL PHYSICAL FEATURES

In the author's view, changes in external appearance only require treatment if they are overtly disfiguring (e.g. pterygium colli) or if they adversely affect the functioning of an organ (e.g. severe ptosis). They should always be treated by particularly skilled doctors. It is quite disheartening to see the disfiguring results of surgery of the pterygium colli when done improperly. Special caution is also recommended since hypertrophic scars are frequently observed in TS, particularly in the area of the neck. Scars from the surgical removal of naevi, which are more frequently seen in an era of more invasive dermatology, may turn out to be cosmetically less desirable than the original moles. Since there is no evidence of a tendency towards malignant degeneration of the common naevi in TS, their removal is mostly a medically questionable activity. Similarly, it is advisable to be cautious when considering surgery on an organ system that shows altered form but functions normally.

During childhood, lymphoedema of hands and—in particular—feet demands little attention, since in most cases with visible oedema at birth, this disappears during childhood. However, in many cases it reappears in adult life. It is for this reason that parents should be advised to buy these children comfortable shoes. In cases with lymphoedema, techniques to improve lymph drainage need to be taught by specialists.

HEARING AND SPEECH

The common dysplasia of the auricles is a cosmetic rather than a functional problem. Otitis media is a very frequent problem, particularly between 1 and 6, with a peak at 3, years of age. In one series, the incidence was found to be as high as 68%, compared with 2–5% in healthy children (Szepunar and Rybak, 1968). The cause is a displacement of the Eustachian tube and impaired ventilation of the middle ear. As a consequence of this, possibly also as the result of inappropriate treatment, and since there are structural abnormalities of the auditory ossicles, impairment of conductive hearing is reported with alarming frequency (Stratton, 1965). Impaired hearing and premature hearing loss based on a defect within the inner ear have been recognized to be frequent in adults (Hultcrantz et al, 1994). In children, impaired hearing negatively influences the development of verbal communication both quantitatively (with regard to sound intensity) and qualitatively (with regard to phonemic discrimination and understanding). Thus, infections of the middle ear need to be treated resolutely whenever they occur. In addition, audiological investigations need to be part of the regular follow-up in TS patients of all ages. Since impaired hearing leads to insufficient speech development and intellectual and psychic impoverishment, its treatment must be appropriate and immediate.

Although verbal abilities are principally normally developed in TS, even patients with normal hearing often have abnormal phonation, with a nasal and squeaking pitch of voice. Since the high-arched palate obstructs nasal air flow and distorts the space of resonance, its correction by orthodontic measures should be attempted.

CARDIOVASCULAR SYSTEM

Cardiovascular abnormalities are a major cause of mortality and morbidity in TS. Apart from coarctation of the aorta (pre-ductal, adult type), bicuspid aortic valve, aortic regurgitation and aortic stenosis, a variety of other congenital malformations have been reported (Mazzanti et al, 1988; Nora et al, 1990). The prevalence of cardiac malformations is about five times higher in patients with the 45,X constitution compared with mosaics. As early as 1959, Haddad and Wilkind drew attention to the high association between webbed neck and coarctation, which points to a pathogenetic link between the two symptoms (Clark, 1984). While overt cardiac malformation is easily recognized and corrected, aortic dissection is an insidious disorder causing fatalities in adult life (Lin et al, 1986). The pathogenetic basis of this is not clear, but there is a higher association with prior coarctation, bicuspid aortic valve and hypertension. In general, the aortic root is found to be wider than in controls (Allen et al, 1986). Blood pressure is often increased even in the absence of cardiac abnormalities, but the prevalence of hypertension in TS is unknown. It is also uncertain whether hypertension is caused by renal or other mechanisms. Given this situation, and in the light of the interdependence of hypertension and aortic dissection, monitoring of blood pressure is mandatory in TS. By the same token, prospective measurements of the aortic root and the ascending aorta by ultrasound are necessary in order to detect the critical point for intervention (at a diameter of the ascending aorta of 5–6 cm: Svensson et al, 1990).

BONES

Aside from occasional congenital malformations of the spine (e.g. block vertebrae) that may need specific orthopaedic treatment, minor malformations of the bones (e.g. Madelung's deformity, shortening of metacarpals or metatarsals) do not cause problems. Abnormalities of the X-ray structure of bones are not associated with an increased tendency towards fractures. Prevention of adult osteoporosis is achieved by timely onset (see below) of continuous oestrogen substitution (see also Chapter 9 in this volume).

METABOLIC DISORDERS

Particularly since the advent of the wider use of GH for the treatment of short stature, there has been a great interest in the metabolism of glucose in TS. In a survey of the literature, Holl and Heinze (1991) found a total frequency of impaired glucose tolerance in 32% (106 out of 326) of women with TS. In addition, Forbes and Engel (1963) reported diabetes mellitus in 6 out of 41 patients aged 30–60 years. Surprisingly, after this publication that suggested a high incidence of diabetes mellitus in TS, only sporadic cases have been reported. Out of the series of 200 adult patients followed by Sybert (1996), only four were suffering from diabetes, and three of these had adult-onset diabetes mellitus and were extremely obese. In our large series of mostly adolescent patients, we have observed only one young adult (aged 32 years) with diabetes. This patient had a history of non-insulin-dependent diabetes mellitus in both parental lines. Based on experience and on the literature, Sybert stated, 'Despite the various abnormalities in glucose tolerance testing that have been reported . . ., I do not believe that adults are at an increased risk for diabetes, either juvenile or adult, outside the risk factor presented by obesity.' Since neither is there an increase in the incidence of diabetes mellitus on high doses of growth hormone (GH) (Wilton, 1994), this statement is likely to be correct. Thus, one should invest time counselling adolescents with TS to avoid the known tendency towards overweight by dietary measures and by stimulating physical activity, rather than by repeatedly investigating children's glucose metabolism (and usually being left with results that are difficult to interpret) (Ranke et al, 1988).

A similar discrepancy between frequently abnormal laboratory findings and infrequency in clinically overt illness exists with regard to thyroid autoimmune disease. While anti-thyroid antibodies are found in about 60% of children with TS (for a review, see Massa et al, 1993), in only 4% is overt hypothyroidism present. The risk is particularly associated with the presence of an iso-X chromosome (de Kerdanet et al, 1994). Thus, careful monitoring of thyroid function and monitoring of thyroid antibodies appears to be well justified during follow-up.

HYPOGONADISM

Substitution of sex steroids

Ovarian failure is a consistent feature of TS, and almost all adolescents and adults require oestrogen treatment for feminization. Although the timing of initiation, the tempo of progression and the mode of oestrogen replacement are still a matter of discussion, there is some consensus about the aspects to be considered.

Age for initiation of therapy

Generally speaking, substitution of oestrogens for feminization needs to be guided by the normal course of puberty in girls. In normal girls, thelarche occurs at a mean age of 10.5 years, with a range of about ±2 years. Puberty progresses from thelarche to menarche within about 2.5 years. The progression of puberty can be monitored by means of breast stages (Tanner) and ultrasonography of the ovaries and uterus, measurement of oestrogen levels having been found to be less helpful. Since pubertal development is paramount for the psychosocial development of any girl, initiation of puberty by means of oestrogen treatment should preferably not be delayed beyond an age of 13 years. At this age, girls with TS usually have a bone age (Greulich and Pyle) of 10.5 years, which is equivalent to the age of normal girls at thelarche. In girls with TS, however, induction of puberty has to be discussed within the context of height development. The timing of onset of oestrogen replacement and the doses of oestrogens given have been discussed in view of their possible beneficial or disadvantageous effects on adult height. The evidence for a rational approach to the problem comes from investigations of patients who enter puberty spontaneously (Massa et al, 1990), from treatment with low oestrogen doses (< 100 ng/kg per day ethinyl oestradiol) at an early age (about or below 11 years) (Ranke et al, 1986; Kastrup, 1988; Neely et al, 1993), and from (conventional) oestrogen replacement at ages of about 12 years and over (Lenko et al, 1979; Sybert, 1984; Ranke and Grauer, 1994). The conclusion from a cautious evaluation of the information given in the literature is that the influence of oestrogens on adult height depends more on the age at onset of exposure to oestrogen than on the dose given. Even low doses of oestrogen given before the age of 12 carry the risk of impairing final height. Oestrogen replacement therapy after an age of approximately 14 years, however, does not appear to affect adult height. No firm recommendation can be given with regard to the influence on adult height when oestrogen replacement is started between the ages of 12 and 14 years. Thus, the introduction of oestrogen replacement in TS at a late-to-normal pubertal age (>13 years) probably does not interfere with adult height.

Modalities of oestrogen replacement

The choice of oestrogen preparation used for feminization during pubertal age depends on availability and the habits within a medical environment. Ethinyl oestradiol, oestradiol valerate, conjugated oestrogens and 17β-oestradiol are commonly used. Oestrogens are usually given orally; trans-dermal application, however, has also been tested. Transdermal application offers the advantage of avoiding the 'first pass' effect, but an appropriate drug is not commercially available and adolescents tend to dislike wearing the patch. It is beyond the scope of this overview to discuss the advantages of different oestrogen preparations. Given the aim of achieving menarche about 2 years after the onset of oestrogen replacement, a recommendation can be made to start with about one quarter of an adult substitution dose, with increments of another quarter adult dose every 6 months. Oestrogens may be given continuously or sequentially (e.g. 3 weeks on, 1 week off). Although some oestrogens may be monitored by measuring their serum levels, monitoring of the progression of the effect may best be done by observing breast stages and uterine volumes. Since the response to oestrogens varies individually, and adequate pubertal progression may occur even on the lower oestrogen doses, the tempo of increase in oestrogens must be individualized. Breast development in TS is usually aesthetically satisfactory. An addition of gestogen preparations (e.g. from day 21 to day 30 of an artificial cycle) is—in accordance with normal pubertal development—not, in our view, mandatory before pubertal stage 4 is reached, which is usually after 1–2 years on oestrogen. When cyclic menstruations occur, regular follow-up by a gynaecologist specializing in adolescents is advisable.

The presence of Y chromosomal material is associated with an increased risk of gonadoblastoma. It is still a matter of discussion whether or not the search for Y chromosomal material using subtle techniques (polymerase chain reaction) should be extended to every case of TS (Page, 1994). However, pelvic ultrasonography should be performed regularly in search of abnormal masses in the region of the ovaries.

FERTILITY

After the 3rd month of gestation in TS, the number of ovarian follicles diminishes dramatically (Stanhope et al, 1993). Although non-functional ('streak') gonads are common, the incidence of residual ovarian tissue may be as high as 30% (Stanhope et al, 1993). In single cases, even spontaneous pregnancies have been reported (Nielsen et al, 1979; Kaneko et al, 1990). Since the techniques of cryopreserving oocytes and ovarian tissue are being refined, there may in future be the possibility of obtaining biological children, in addition to embryo transfer after in vitro fertilization of a donor oocyte (Van Steirteghem et al, 1992; Gosden et al, 1994). Although there are still open medical and ethical questions regarding this approach, counselling of adolescents along these lines should give girls with TS a more positive outlook on life.

GROWTH PROBLEMS

Natural growth in TS

Short stature is the most constant feature in TS. It is present in patients with the 45,X karyotype—which is found in about 50–60% of all patients—and in patients with other chromosomal abnormalities. Growth in TS can be schematically divided into four phases:

1   There is intrauterine growth retardation. In children born near term, the average length is approximately 3 cm less than in normal children.
2   There is near-to-normal growth during infancy and early childhood.
3   There is considerable relative loss of height during childhood. From about 3 to 12 years of age, children with TS lose about 15 cm in height compared with normal girls.
4   Since puberty does not occur, there is no pubertal growth spurt and the total growth phase is prolonged. However, there is only a minor (approximately 5 cm) additional relative loss of height during this phase, which has probably very little to do with the absence of puberty (Massa et al, 1990).

The reported adult height varies among publications (for a review, see Ranke and Grauer, 1994). The mean adult stature in TS of Caucasian origin is approximately 142–147 cm. When comparing reports about the adult height in TS from different ethnic backgrounds, there appears to be a difference of 20 cm between mean normal female adult height and adult height in TS within a given population. The variability of height is similar in quantity to that observed in the normal population. There is a positive correlation between the adult height reached and parental height (Ranke and Grauer, 1994).

Although the general pattern of growth is well described, and disease-specific standards (including growth charts) have been devised for height (Lyon et al, 1985; Ranke et al, 1988) and height velocity (Ranke et al, 1988, 1991), the issue of whether or not patients with different karyotypes grow in an identical or different mode is still not finally settled.

Several attempts are being made to predict adult height in individuals more accurately (Frane et al, 1990; Joss, 1991; Naeraa et al, 1991). At present, the most widely accepted model is to plot the growth of an individual girl with TS on a TS-specific growth chart and to extend this line following the individual percentile to a 'projected final height'. The validity of this approach to predicting adult height is supported by empirical evidence (Lyon et al, 1985). In the author's view, this appears to be quite a sound approach. It assumes that childhood growth in TS follows the channel of targetted height, and that individual influences on a child's growth (e.g. parental height) are already expressed within the deviation of height from the disease-specific mean for a given age. The existence of disease-specific norms for height and the ability to predict individual adult height provide the basis for attempts to treat short stature in TS.

Rationale for growth-promoting therapies

The reason for short stature in TS is at present unknown. Most investigators believe that a disorder at the growth tissue level is responsible for short stature. Some, however, favour the idea that hormones may—at least partially—be a cause. In particular, a disorder of the GH–insulin-like growth factor (IGF) axis has been discussed. There is no doubt that the response of GH to provocative tests is often poor, and that the amount of GH secreted spontaneously is frequently subnormal. At pubertal age, spontaneously secreted GH is definitely below the levels found in normal girls during puberty (Buchanan et al, 1987; Ranke et al, 1987). Likewise, low or subnormal IGF-I levels have been found during that period (Cuttler et al, 1985; Ross et al, 1985; Ranke et al, 1987). This, however, has been attributed to the absence of oestrogen and to mild obesity, since the conditions can be reversed by oestrogen application and/or reduction in weight (Schober et al, 1987). The serum levels of the GH-dependent IGF-binding protein (IGFBP-3), which are highly correlated with spontaneous GH secretion, have been found to be within the normal range (Ranke et al, 1989). It has also been shown that age-matched girls, with or without low GH secretion, grow at similar rates with or without exogenous GH (Massa et al, 1990). Thus, there is no convincing evidence that GH deficiency is involved in the pathogenesis of the growth disorder in TS, even though a recent study showing heterogeneity in circulating forms of GH (Blethen et al, 1994) has given new corroboration to the opposing view.

Treatment with GH

When pituitary human GH first became available, a few patients with TS were treated with it (Hutchings, 1965; Tzagournis, 1969). The results of these trials were largely disappointing. With the availability of abundant amounts of GH produced by the recombinant technique, it has been possible to conduct carefully designed studies with the aim of re-evaluating this approach. The prototype of all recent studies is the one of the Genentech Study Group, of which successive reports have been published (Rosenfeld et al, 1992). In this study, a representative cohort of girls with TS was treated with GH. Out of the original 65 patients entering the study at a mean age of 9.3 years, 30 have discontinued therapy after a mean duration of treatment of 54 months and at a mean age of 16.7 years. The patients received a weekly GH dose of approximately 1.0 IU/kg body weight (BW) (0.375 mg/kg BW), sometimes combined with oxandrolone (0.125–0.065 mg/kg BW per day). The gain above projected adult height averaged 8.1 cm, with many of the patients still growing. By now, the results of long-term follow-up of a number of large collaborative studies have been or are about to be published (Heinrichs et al, 1996; Massa et al, 1996; Nilsson et al, 1996; Ranke et al, 1996; Rochiccioli and Chaussain, 1996; Stahnke et al, 1996; Takano et al, 1996). In addition, meta-analyses of large cohorts of patients within multicentric/multinational studies have been conducted, allowing the definition of those factors influencing the outcome of GH treatment (Hintz et al, 1996; Ranke et al, 1996).

Without aiming to discuss individually the details of the study designs, the diffent methodologies to evaluate the growth response and the results of each of the studies, the general lessons taught by the studies will be briefly outlined.

1. GH given in higher than substitutive doses (e.g. 0.7–1.5 IU/kg per week, given as equal daily subcutaneous injections) is able to increase adult height in TS. Many patients treated have surpassed 150 cm, a socially acceptable height for adult women.
2. The gain in height is positively correlated to the dose applied.
3. Most gain is observed during the first 3 years of treatment.
4. The individual response is highly variable and so far not predictable.
5. The statural outcome is negatively correlated with the age at onset of treatment with GH. Since there is so far only a little experience with treatment before an age of 7 years, nothing can be said about the optimal age for onset of GH treatment in younger children.
6. The anabolic steroid oxandrolone given in conjunction with GH (0.0625–0.05 mg/kg per day orally) increases the tempo of growth, thus shortening the overall duration of GH treatment to reach final height. Oxandrolone most probably also adds to the total gain in height. Its mechanism of action, however, is still unclear.
7. There is no evidence that there is a place for oestrogens as a therapy to increase adult height.
8. Since there are still many questions concerning GH (with or without oxandrolone and/or oestrogens), patients should be followed within

studies and surveys. This also applies in countries in which GH is approved by health authorities and paid for by third parties (e.g. health insurances).

Risks of growth-promoting therapy

The potential risks of growth-promoting therapies are posed by (a) specific factors related to TS, (b) specific side-effects of the drugs used, (c) the dosage and duration of the drugs used, and (d) a combination of these factors. In spite of the risk potential of GH therapy with supraphysiological doses, the observed incidence of adverse events in TS is not essentially different from that seen in idiopathic GH deficiency (Wilton, 1994). In particular, the incidence of overt non-insulin dependent diabetes mellitus was not increased. At present, we know rather little about the spontaneous outcome of patients, since there are only insufficient data available on TS in adult life. Impaired glucose tolerance and a tendency towards high blood pressure (even without cardiac failure) are well-documented abnormalities in TS (for a review, see Chiumello et al, 1991; Wilson et al, 1988). High doses of GH may increase the risk of developing diabetes mellitus. Although recent studies have shown that the negative effects of GH on glucose tolerance were transient (Wilson et al, 1988; Sippell et al, 1991; Stahnke et al, 1991), the long-term risks cannot be predicted. Oxandrolone has been in use for decades and appears to be rather safe when given in low doses. However, its potential hazards when given over long periods of time are by no means established. Since the dose risk potential may be age-dependent, care must be taken when treating younger patients.

PSYCHOSOCIAL AND INTELLECTUAL ASPECTS

The issues of psychosocial development, intellectual performance and social integration of TS patients have drawn much attention. A review of the related scientific activities is beyond the scope of this article. In general, it is probably fair to state that there are no or only minor primary intellectual deficits in TS. In particular, verbal abilities have been reported to be normal, while impairment of visual–spatial and spatial–perceptual abilities has been described (Rovet, 1971; McCauley et al, 1986; Netley and Rovet, 1992). Thus, it is mandatory to advise parents from the moment of the diagnosis to raise their children as any normal child, to make the same demands and to give the same support. It is an over-protective attitude combined with inappropriate challenges that may lead to psychosocial infantilism in children and adults with TS.

SUMMARY

The care for patients with TS needs to be comprehensive, addressing specific problems in relation to their developmental perspective. This care needs a long-term strategy involving competent specialists for 'managing' specific questions and also a generalist's approach of emphatic guidance. Given this, TS is a disorder with an optimistic lifetime perspective.

REFERENCES

Albertsson-Wikland K & Ranke MB (eds) (1995) *Turner Syndrome—in a Life-span Perspective.* Amsterdam: Elsevier.

Allen DB, Hendricks SA & Levy JM (1986) Aortic dilatation in Turner syndrome. *Journal of Pediatrics* 109: 302.

Blethen SL, Albertsson-Wikland K, Faklis EJ & Chasalow FI (1994) Circulating growth hormone isoforms in girls with Turner's syndrome. *Journal of Clinical Endocrinology and Metabolism* 78: 1439–1443.

Buchanan CR, Law CM & Milner RDG (1987) Growth hormone in short, slowly growing children and those with Turner's syndrome. *Archives of Disease in Childhood* 62: 912–916.

Chiumello G, Bognetti E, Bonfanti R et al (1991) Glucose metabolism in Turner syndrome. In Ranke MB & Rosenfeld RG (eds) *Turner Syndrome: Growth Promoting Therapies*, pp 47–49. Amsterdam: Excerpta Medica, Elsevier.

Clark EB (1984) Neck web and congenital heart defects: a pathogenetic association in 45,XO Turner syndrome? *Teratology* 29: 355.

Cuttler L, Van Vliet G, Conte FA et al (1985) Somatomedin-C levels in children and adolescents with gonadal dysgenesis: differences from age-matched normal females and effect of chronic estrogen replacement therapy. *Journal of Clinical Endocrinology and Metabolism* 60: 1087–1092.

Forbes AP & Engel E (1963) The high incidence of diabetes mellitus in 41 patients with gonadal dysgenesis and their close relatives. *Metabolism* 12: 428–439.

Frane JW, Sherman BW and the Genentech Collaborative Group (1990) Predicted adult height in Turner syndrome. In Rosenfeld RG & Grumbach MM (eds) *Turner Syndrome*, pp 393–403. New York: Marcel Dekker.

Gosden RG, Baird DT, Wade JC & Webb R (1994) Restoration of fertility to oophorectomized sheep by ovarian autografts stored at −196 (degrees). *Human Reproduction* 9: 597–603.

Heinrichs C, De Schepper J, Thomas M et al (1996) Final height in 46 girls with Turner's syndrome treated with growth hormone in Belgium: evaluation of height recovery and predictive factors. In Albertsson-Wikland K & Ranke MB (eds) *Turner Syndrome—A Life Time Perspective.* Amsterdam: Elsevier (in press).

Hibi I & Takano K (eds) (1993) *Basic and Clinical Approach to Turner syndrome.* Amsterdam: Elsevier.

Hibi I, Tanae A, Tanaka T et al (1991) Spontaneous puberty in Turner Syndrome: its incidence, influence on final height and endocrinological features. In Ranke MB & Rosenfeld RG (eds) *Turner Syndrome: Growth Promoting Therapies*, pp 75–81. Amsterdam: Excerpta Medica, Elsevier.

Hintz RL, Attie KM, Compton PG & Rosenfeld RG (1996) Multifactorial studies of GH treatment of Turner syndrome: the Genentech National Cooperative Growth Study. In Albertsson-Wikland K & Ranke MB (eds) *Turner Syndrome—A Life Time Perspective.* Amsterdam: Elsevier (in press).

Holl RW & Heinze E (1991) Gestörte Glukosetoleranz und Diabetes mellitus beim Ullrich–Turner–Syndrom. *Monatsschrift Kinderheilkunde* 139: 676–680.

Hultcrantz M, Sylven L & Borg E (1994) Ear and hearing problems in 44 middle-aged women with Turner syndrome. *Hearing Research* 76: 127–132.

Hutchings J, Escamilla R, Li C & Forsham P (1965) Li human growth hormone administration in gonadal dysgenesis. *American Journal of Diseases of Childhood* 109: 312–318.

Joss E (1991) Evaluation of hormonal treatment on linear growth and skeletal maturation; methods of predicting final height in Turner syndrome. In Ranke MB & Rosenfeld RG (eds) *Turner Syndrome: Growth Promoting Therapies*, pp 83–88. Amsterdam: Excerpta Medica, Elsevier.

Kaneko N, Kawagoe S & Hizoi M (1990) Turner's syndrome review of the literature with reference to a successful pregnancy outcome. *Gynecologic and Obstetric Investigation* 29: 81–87.

Kastrup KW (1988) Oestrogen therapy in Turner's syndrome. *Acta Paediatrica Scandinavica* 343 (supplement): 43–46.

Kerdanet M de, Lucas J, Lemee F & Lecornu M (1994) Turner's syndrome with x-isochromosome and Hashimoto's thyroiditis. *Clinical Endocrinology* **41:** 673–676.

Lenko HL, Perheentuppa J & Soederholm A (1979) Growth in Turner's syndrome: spontaneous and fluoxymestrone stimulated. *Acta Paediatrica Scandinavica* **277 (supplement):** 57–63.

Lin AE, Lippe BM, Geffner ME et al (1986) Aortic dilatation, dissection, and rupture in patients with Turner syndrome. *Journal of Pediatrics* **109:** 820.

Lippe BM (1991) Turner syndrome. *Endocrinology and Metabolism Clinics of North America* **20:** 121–152.

Lyon AJ, Preece MA & Grant DB (1985) Growth curve for girls with Turner's syndrome. *Archives of Disease in Childhood* **60:** 932–935.

Massa G, Vanderscheuren-Lodeweyckx M & Malvaux P (1990) Linear growth in patients with Turner syndrome: influence of spontaneous puberty and parental height. *European Journal of Pediatrics* **149:** 246–250.

McCauley E, Ito J & Kay T (1986) Psychosocial functioning in girls with the Turner's syndrome and short stature: social skills, behavior problems, and self concept. *Journal of the American Academy for Child Psychology* **25:** 105–110.

Massa G, de Zegher F & Vanderscheuren-Lodeweyckx M (1993) Thyroid function in Turner syndrome. In Hibi I & Takano K (eds) *Basic and Clinical Approach to Turner Syndrome*, pp 129–135. Amsterdam: Elsevier.

Massa G, Van den Broeck J, Attanasio A & Wit JM, on behalf of the Lilly European Turner Study Group (1996) Final height results of the Lilly European Turner Study. In Albertsson-Wikland K & Ranke MB (eds) *Turner Syndrome—A Life Time Perspective*. Amsterdam: Elsevier.

Mazzanti L, Prandstraller D, Tassinari D et al (1988) Heart disease in Turner syndrome. *Helvetica Paediatrica Acta* **43:** 25.

Naeraa RW, Eiken M, Legarth EG & Nielsen J (1991) Spontaneous growth, final height and prediction of final height in Turner syndrome. In Ranke MB & Rosenfeld RG (eds) *Turner Syndrome: Growth Promoting Therapies*, pp 113–116. Amsterdam: Excerpta Medica, Elsevier.

Neely EE, Rosenfeld RG and the Gynex Cooperative Study Group (1993) First year results of a randomized, placebo-controlled trial of low-dose ethinyl-estradiol for feminization during growth hormone therapy for Turner syndrome. *Pediatric Research* **33:** 89 (abstract).

Netley C & Rovet J (1992) Atypical hemispheric lateralization in Turner syndrome subjects. *Cortex* **18:** 377–384.

Nielsen J, Sillesen I & Hansen KB (1979) Fertility in women with Turner's syndrome. Case report and review of the literature. *British Journal of Obstetrics and Gynaecology* **86:** 833–835.

Nilsson KO, Albertsson-Wikland K, Alm J et al (1996) Growth promoting treatment in girls with Turner syndrome: final height results according to three different Turner syndrome standards. In Albertsson-Wikland K & Ranke MB (eds) *Turner Syndrome—A Life Time Perspective*. Amsterdam: Elsevier.

Nora JJ, Torres FG, Sinha AK & McNamara DG (1990) Characteristic cardiovascular abnormalities of X0 Turner syndrome, XX and XY phenotype and X0/XX Turner mosaic. *American Journal of Cardiology* **25:** 639.

Page DC (1994) Y-chromosomal sequences in Turner's syndrome and risk of gonadoblastoma and virilisation. *Lancet* **343:** 240–242.

Ranke MB (1989) *An Introduction to Turner's Syndrome*. Oxford: Oxford Clinical Communications.

Ranke MB & Grauer ML (1994) Adult height in Turner syndrome: results of a multinational survey 1993. *Hormone Research* **42:** 90–94.

Ranke MB & Rosenfeld RG (eds) (1991) *Turner Syndrome: Growth Promoting Therapies*. Amsterdam: Excerpta Medica, Elsevier.

Ranke MB, Blum WF & Frisch H (1989) The acid-stable subunit of insulin-like growth factor binding protein (IGFBP-3) in disorders of growth. In Drop SLS & Hintz RL (eds) *Insulin-like Growth Factor Binding Proteins*, pp 103–112. Amsterdam: Excerpta Medica, Elsevier.

Ranke MB, Stubbe P, Majewski F & Bierich JR (1988) Spontaneous growth in Turner's syndrome. *Acta Paediatrica Scandinavica* **343 (supplement):** 22–30.

Ranke MB, Haug F, Blum WF et al (1986) Effect on growth of patients with Turner's syndrome treated with low estrogen doses. *Acta Endocrinologica* **276 (supplement):** 153–156.

Ranke MB, Blum WF, Haug F et al (1987) Growth hormone, somatomedin levels and growth regulation in Turner's syndrome. *Acta Endocrinologica* **116:** 305–313.

Ranke MB, Chavez-Mayer H, Blank B et al (1991) Spontaneous growth and bone age development in Turner syndrome—results of a multicentric study 1990. In Ranke MB & Rosenfeld RG (eds)

Turner Syndrome: Growth Promoting Therapies, pp 101–106. Amsterdam: Excerpta Medica, Elsevier.

Ranke MB, Price DA, Maes M et al (1995) for the International Board of the Kabi International Growth Study (KIGS) 1995.

Rochiccioli P & Chaussain JL (1996) Final height in patients with Turner syndrome treated with growth hormone (N=117). In Albertsson-Wikland K & Ranke MB (eds) *Turner Syndrome—A Life Time Perspective*. Amsterdam: Elsevier (in press).

Rosenfeld RG & Grumbach MM (eds) (1990) *Turner Syndrome*. New York: Marcel Dekker.

Rosenfeld RG, Frane J, Attie KM et al (1992) Six year results of a randomized, prospective trial of human growth hormone and oxandrolone in Turner syndrome. *Journal of Pediatrics* **121:** 49–55.

Ross JL, Long LM, Loriaux LD & Cutler GB (1985) Growth hormone secretory dynamics in Turner syndrome. *Journal of Pediatrics* **106:** 202–206.

Rovet JF (1971) The cognitive and neuropsychological characteristics of females with Turner syndrome. In Bender B & Berch D (eds) *Sex Chromosome Abnormalities and Behavior: Psychological Studies*, pp 39–77. Boulder, Colorado: Westview Press.

Schober E, Frisch H, Waldhauser F & Biegelmayer CH (1987) Influence of estrogen administration on growth hormone stimulation in patients with Turner's syndrome. *Acta Endocrinologica* **283 (supplement):** 175–176.

Sippell WG, Partsch CJ & Steinkamp H (1991) Biosynthetic growth hormone (Genotropin) therapy in girls with the Ullrich–Turner syndrome (UTS). In Ranke MB & Rosenfeld RG (eds) *Turner Syndrome: Growth Promoting Therapies*, pp 237–240. Amsterdam: Excerpta Medica, Elsevier.

Stahnke N, Stubbe P, Keller E, Zeisel HJ and the Serono Study Group Hamburg (1991) Effects and side effects of GH plus oxandrolone in Turner syndrome. In Ranke MB and Rosenfeld RG (eds) *Turner Syndrome: Growth Promoting Therapies*, pp 241–248. Amsterdam: Excerpta Medica, Elsevier.

Stahnke N, Attanasio A, van den Broeck J et al (1996) GH treatment studies to final height in girls with Turner syndrome—the German experience. In Albertsson-Wikland K & Ranke MB (eds) *Turner Syndrome—A Life Time Perspective*. Amsterdam: Elsevier (in press).

Stanhope R, Massarano A & Brook CGD (1993) The natural course of ovarian demise in Turner syndrome. In Hibi I & Takano K (eds) *Basic and Clinical Approach to Turner Syndrome*, pp 93–100. Amsterdam: Excerpta Medica, Elsevier.

Stratton HJM (1965) Gonadal dysgenesis and the ears. *Journal of Laryngology and Otology* **79:** 343.

Svensson LG, Crawford ES, Hess KR et al (1990) Dissection of the aorta and dissecting aortic aneurysma: improving early and long-term surgical results. *Circulation* **82 (supplement IV):** 24–38.

Sybert VP (1984) Adult height in Turner Syndrome with and without androgen therapy. *Journal of Pediatrics* **104:** 365–369

Sybert VP (1996) The adult patient with Turner syndrome. In Albertsson-Wikland K & Ranke MB (eds) *Turner Syndrome—A Life Time Perspective*. Amsterdam: Elsevier (in press).

Szepunar J & Rybak M (1968) Middle ear disease in Turner's syndrome. *Archives of Otolaryngology—Head and Neck Surgery* **87:** 34.

Takano K, Ogawa M, Okada Y et al (1996) In Albertsson-Wikland K & Ranke MB (eds) *Turner Syndrome—A Life Time Perspective*. Amsterdam: Elsevier (in press).

Tzagournis M (1969) Response to long-term administration of human growth hormone in Turner's syndrome. *Journal of the American Medical Association* **210:** 2373–2376.

Van Steirteghem AC, Pados G, Devroey P et al (1992) Oocyte donation for genetic indications. *Reproduction Fertility and Development* **4:** 681–688.

Werther G, Dietsch S, for the Australasian Paediatric Endocrine Group (1996) Multi-centre trial of synthetic growth hormone and low dose oestrogen in Turner syndrome. In Albertsson-Wikland K & Ranke MB (eds) *Turner Syndrome—A Life Time Perspective*. Amsterdam: Elsevier (in press).

Wilson DM, Frane J, Sherman B et al (1988) Carbohydrate and lipid metabolism in Turner syndrome: effect of therapy with growth hormone, oxandrolone, and a combination of both. *Journal of Pediatrics* **112:** 210–217.

Wilton P (1994) Adverse events during growth hormone treatment: 5 years' experience in the Kabi International Growth Study. In Ranke MB & Gunnarsson R (eds) *Progress in Growth Hormone Therapy—5 Years of KIGS*, pp 291–307. Mannheim: J&J Verlag.

6

Glucocorticoids and growth

BURKHARD TÖNSHOFF
CHRISTIAN JUX
OTTO MEHLS

Glucocorticoid therapy in pharmacological doses is an essential treatment modality in various chronic inflammatory and immune-mediated diseases in childhood. In addition, glucocorticoids are needed for immuno-suppression after organ transplantation. Long-term, high-dose gluco-corticoid medication in children inevitably leads to growth failure and protein catabolism. Recent evidence indicates that these side-effects are partially mediated by alterations of the somatotrophic hormone axis. This review summarizes (a) the current knowledge about the interference of glucocorticoids with the production and action of growth hormone (GH) and insulin-like growth factors (IGFs), (b) describes the optimization of glucocorticoid therapy in chronic paediatric diseases, such as bronchial asthma, atopic eczema, juvenile chronic arthritis, inflammatory bowel disease and nephrotic syndrome, and in patients post-renal transplantation, (c) discusses the therapeutic potential of the new glucocorticoid analogue deflazacort, and (d) presents the current status of concomitant anabolic treatment with recombinant human (rh) GH and IGF-I for glucocorticoid-induced growth failure.

PATHOPHYSIOLOGY OF GLUCOCORTICOID/GH INTERACTIONS

The growth-inhibiting effects of glucocorticoids are multifactorial and involve alterations in the secretory profiles of GH, inhibition of IGF-I bioactivity by the production of inhibitors, alterations in IGF-binding protein concentration and direct effects on the local regulation of growth factors and skeletal tissue matrix (Table 1).

Biphasic effect of glucocorticoids on GH secretion

While short-term glucocorticoid administration stimulates GH secretion (Casanueva et al, 1990; Veldhuis et al, 1992), high-dose, long-term gluco-corticoid treatment suppresses spontaneous GH secretion in some, but not

Baillière's Clinical Paediatrics—
Vol. 4, No. 2, May 1996
ISBN 0–7020–2180–6
0963–6714/96/020309 + 24 $12.00/00

Table 1. Interference of long-term, high-dose glucocorticoid treatment with the integrity of the somatotrophic hormone axis.

Organ	Effect of glucocorticoids
Hypothalamus	Somatostatin tone ↑
Hypophysis	GH secretion ↓
Liver	GH-induced IGF-I mRNA ↓
Circulation	IGF-I levels normal or ↑
	Induction of IGF inhibitors
	IGFBP-2 ↑
Epiphyseal growth plate	Cell proliferation ↓
	Matrix production ↓
	Paracrine IGF-I secretion ↓
	GH and type I IGF receptor ↓

all, individuals. Several studies performed in men (Wehrenberg et al, 1990) have shown that the inhibitory effect of glucocorticoids on GH secretion in vivo are due to enhancement of hypothalamic somatostatin release. Recent data indicate that arginine infusion, by inhibition of endogenous hypothalamic somatostatin tone, is able to normalize the GH response to GH-releasing hormone in adult patients receiving chronic daily immunosuppressive glucocorticoid therapy (Giustina et al, 1992). In peri-pubertal children with renal transplants, a significant inverse relationship between the daily dose of glucocorticoids and the peak amplitude or mean levels of GH was noted, whereas the GH pulse frequency was not changed (Schaefer et al, 1991); similar results were obtained in rats during experimental methylprednisolone treatment (Kovacs et al, 1991). Indeed, a significant number of children with renal transplants appear to have glucocorticoid-induced GH hyposecretion; in one study, 8 out of 17 adolescents with short stature on alternate-day steroids had decreased secretion of GH (Rees et al, 1988b). The dose of glucocorticoids and the time period required to suppress GH secretion under clinical conditions are not known.

GH receptor

There is recent experimental evidence that long-term exposure to pharmacological doses of glucocorticoids suppresses GH receptor expression, at least in the liver. While adrenalectomy does not appear to affect hepatic GH receptor binding and plasma levels of GH-binding protein (GHBP) in the rat, these parameters were markedly reduced in a dose-dependent fashion by dexamethasone treatment, which also compromised growth rate in these otherwise normal animals (Gabrielsson et al, 1995). These depressive effects on GH receptor mRNA levels were found irrespective of whether dexamethasone, methylprednisolone or corticosterone was used. Under clinical conditions, GH receptor status can be assessed by determination of the high-affinity GHBP, which is derived from the extracellular domain of the GH receptor by proteolytic cleavage. In patients on glucocorticoids post-renal transplantation, we observed a significant reduction of circulating GHBP levels compared with age-matched controls (Tönshoff and Mehls, 1994). These clinical data confirm the experimental concept that long-term exposure to glucocorticoids might reduce the tissue sensitivity to GH by a downregulation of the GH receptor.

IGFs and IGF-binding proteins

If chronic glucocorticoid treatment suppresses spontaneous GH secretion, one would expect a decrease of circulating IGF-I levels, which are mainly regulated by circulating GH and the nutritional status. However, circulating immunoreactive IGF-I levels in glucocorticoid-treated children with renal transplants are normal (Tönshoff et al, 1993). In patients with chronic endogenous glucocorticoid excess, IGF-I levels are elevated (Bang et al, 1993). Lower-normal range IGF-I levels in one study (Aitman et al, 1989) may be explained by interference of IGF binding proteins (IGFBPs) in the IGF-I radio-immunoassay, because prior separation by acid size chromatography was not performed.

Under experimental conditions, the GH-induced rise in serum IGF-I in hypophysectomized rats was significantly inhibited by high doses of dexamethasone (Luo and Murphy, 1989). Concomitantly, the GH-induced IGF-I mRNA content in liver, tibia, lung and kidney was inhibited by dexamethasone pre-treatment. There was also a reduction of the hepatic IGF-I mRNA abundance in dexamethasone-treated intact rats. The authors suggested two possible explanations: (1) hepatic IGF-I mRNA is not translated into protein, or (2) glucocorticoids alter the translation, synthesis and secretion of IGF-I in such a way that the IGF-I mRNA abundance no longer reflects IGF-I protein synthesis.

Although glucocorticoids do not consistently reduce circulating immunoreactive IGF-I levels under clinical conditions, they inhibit IGF bio-activity. When methylprednisolone 2 mg/kg body weight was given as an intravenous bolus to children with the nephrotic syndrome, an abrupt decrease in serum IGF activity was noted, which remained low for 24 hours (Elders et al, 1975). An almost 50% reduction in IGF activity was noted in adults given a single 16 mg dose of prednisone, without any significant change in immunoreactive IGF-I levels (Unterman and Phillips, 1985). Low-dose prednisone treatment at a dose of about 0.5 mg/kg per day decreases serum IGF activity in children with a variety of disorders (Green et al, 1978). The reduced IGF activity is not explained by low concentrations of circulating IGF-I, because a dose of prednisone sufficient to lower circulating IGF activity did not reduce serum IGF-I concentrations (Unterman and Phillips, 1985). Hence, glucocorticoid excess apparently does not impair immunoreactive IGF-I levels, but rather antagonizes the action of IGF by a direct and/or indirect mechanism, possibly by the production of IGF inhibitors. These IGF inhibitors, with a molecular weight of 12–20 kDa, which differed from IGFBPs in several ways, have, however, not been further characterized.

The action and metabolism of IGFs are modulated by specific high-affinity IGFBPs, which bind approximately 99% of circulating IGF. Chronic endogenous glucocorticoid excess in patients with Cushing's syndrome was associated with a slight increase of IGFBP-3 in proportion to the increased IGF-I levels, normal IGFBP-1 levels and clearly elevated IGFBP-2 levels (Bang et al, 1993). The molecular weight forms of IGF-I and IGFBP-3 in Cushing's syndrome serum did not differ from those displayed by normal serum. This study suggests a possible role for IGFBP-2 as an IGF inhibitor during glucocorticoid excess. Miell et al (1993) investigated the effect of short-term glucocorticoid treatment with dexamethasone, 4 mg per day for 4 days, in six healthy volunteers. Treatment nearly doubled the serum IGF-I concentration, which was explained by a slight concomitant increase of serum IGFBP-3 levels. Concomitantly, the serum concentration of IGFBP-2 decreased, and the normal increase in the concentration of IGFBP-1 during the night was diminished. Hence, the effect of glucocorticoids on serum IGFBP-2 levels may be dependent on the duration of exposure.

Growth suppression at the cellular level

Some children with growth failure under chronic glucocorticoid therapy have normal serum GH and IGF-I levels. These findings point to some degree of end-organ insensitivity responsible for the growth disturbance. For more than a decade, cell cultures of growth plate chondrocytes and various kinds of bone-related cell have provided a helpful model to study the mechanisms of steroid effects in peripheral tissue.

According to the 'dual-effector theory', GH renders chondrocyte precursor cells in the germinal layer of the growth plate IGF-I-responsive by expressing type 1 IGF receptors on cell surfaces. In addition to the endocrine IGF-I production in the liver, GH promotes local IGF-I gene expression and IGF-I secretion, which in turn causes clonal expansion of chondrocytes in the proliferative cell layer of the growth plate by auto- and paracrine mechanisms (Green et al, 1985; Isaksson et al, 1987). Longitudinal bone growth is the result of chondrocyte proliferation and subsequent enchondral ossification in the epiphyseal growth plates. Glucocorticoids interfere with chondrocyte growth and enchondral bone formation in various ways. They have been shown to inhibit sulphatation of cartilage matrix, as well as mineralization and formation of new bone (Silbermann and Maor, 1978). In recent experiments using the model of cultured epiphyseal chondrocytes, dexamethasone dose- and time-dependently decreased DNA synthesis and cell proliferation through reduction of GH receptor expression and inhibition of homologous up-regulation of both the GH- and the IGF-I receptor. Furthermore, glucocorticoids significantly lowered paracrine IGF-I secretion. These in vitro effects could at least partially be counterbalanced by addition of GH in supraphysiological doses into the cell culture medium (Figure 1) (Robinson et al, 1995; Jux et al, 1996). It should be noted, however, that other growth factors, such as calciotrophic hormones, also strongly influence epiphyseal cell growth and exhibit numerous interactions with both the somatotrophic hormone axis and glucocorticoids (Klaus et al, 1994).

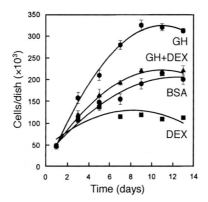

Figure 1. Effect of dexamethasone (DEX) on basal and GH-mediated proliferation of freshly isolated growth plate chondrocytes. The cells were incubated in BSA (●), DEX (10^{-7}M) (■), GH (40 ng/ml) (●), or a combination of DEX and GH (▲). Reproduced from Robinson et al (1995, *Acta Paediatrica* **411 (supplement):** 81–86) with permission.

At present, little is known about the precise mechanism whereby glucocorticoids regulate the gene activity that eventually leads to growth disturbance. It is generally believed that glucocorticoids exert their genomic effects after cytosolic binding to specific receptors. Once conformational changes and translocation to the nucleus have occurred, the complexes bind to DNA at specific consensus sites, termed glucocorticoid response elements, on the upstream promoter sequence of steroid-responsive genes. Some current research is focusing on the inhibition of GH-induced tyrosyl phosphorylation of the GH receptor and various kinases and transcription factors by glucocorticoids (Slootweg et al, 1991; King and Carter-Su, 1995).

OPTIMIZATION OF GLUCOCORTICOID THERAPY IN CHRONIC PAEDIATRIC DISEASES

Bronchial asthma

Influence of the underlying chronic disorder

As in other states of chronic disease, asthma itself influences the normal growth pattern. In 1868, Salter first described that patients with young onset of asthma are '*generally* below the average height. Some asthmatics, however … have nothing whatever the matter with their appearance'. Later clinical investigation showed that the same holds true for other allergic diseases, such as allergic rhinitis only. Furthermore, only a weak association between the clinical severity of the underlying pathology (reflected by efficacy of treatment and symptom control) and pre-pubertal growth retardation was observed.

In a detailed, long-term prospective study, 45% of 66 children with chronic perennial asthma developed transient growth retardation due to delayed puberty in association with a prolonged and deepened nadir of pre-pubertal growth velocity, starting at the age of about 10 years. For that life-span, a three-fold higher prevalence of short stature could be estimated for asthmatic children in comparison with the overall population. Although there was a male preponderance in the total number of cases, onset of puberty was equally and significantly delayed for both sexes. These observations were noted to be independent of severity of asthma as well as its treatment. However, once the pubertal growth spurt started in these children, their adult height was fully achieved by compensatory catch-up growth (Balfour-Lynn, 1986). Thus growth failure due to asthma itself should be regarded as a maturational problem with a benign long-term prognosis.

Influence of glucocorticoid medication: systemic versus inhalational therapy

Glucocorticoids are still the most effective therapy available in the treatment of asthma. Stunting of growth has been described as a dose- and duration-dependent side-effect since its introduction as anti-asthmatic therapy in children (Blodgett et al, 1956). In one of the early studies, the heights of 8% (4 out of 49) of young asthmatics who had not yet received steroids were 2 standard deviations below the mean. However, 15% (24 out of 158) of children on oral, intermittent (less than 50% of days per year) and 33% (31 out of 95) on continuous (no interruptions longer than 2 weeks) corticosteroid therapy fell into this group (Falliers et al, 1963). While there is general agreement on the growth-retarding effect in children with asthma on continuous oral glucocorticoid medication, there has been an ongoing controversy regarding the impact of inhaled corticosteroid therapy on linear growth.

Balfour-Lynn (1986), in his long-term study, found no adverse effect on growth in pre-pubertal children receiving inhaled beclomethasone diproprionate (BDP) in a dose of up to 600 µg per day or up to 400 µg per day during puberty. In fact, it is no paradox that glucocorticoids, while having intrinsic growth-stunting properties, can at the same time promote growth in the young by controlling the disease process and increasing energy intake, an observation made earlier by Cohen and Abram (1948). On the assumption that symptoms of chronic asthma are well controlled by treatment, even dosages of up to 1600 µg per day BDP or budesonide (BUD) in the pre-pubertal age group did not impair growth velocity over a follow-up period of up to 5 years (Ninan and Russell, 1992). However, when the asthma was poorly controlled, the height velocity standard deviation score (SDS) decreased to −1.55, both before and after starting inhaled corticosteroid therapy.

The growth-preserving safety of inhaled corticosteroid therapy is also confirmed by a recent meta-analysis of 21 studies including 810 asthmatic children (Allen et al, 1994). There was a significant but weak tendency for corticosteroid treatment in general to be associated with growth impairment. More specifically, prednisone and other oral corticosteroids were significantly associated with growth impairment, whereas inhaled BDP showed a significant tendency to be associated with attaining normal height. Adverse effects of inhaled corticosteroid therapy on growth appeared more likely after 11 years of age, a finding in accordance with delayed puberty. No statistical evidence was found for inhalative corticosteroid therapy to be associated with growth impairment at a higher dosage, for longer therapy duration or in more severe asthma. Although these data are reassuring, careful and close monitoring of growth is mandatory in children on long-term inhaled corticosteroid therapy, since in individual cases growth depression can be severe (Hollman and Allen, 1988).

General therapeutic guidelines for minimizing growth-depressing side-effects of glucocorticoids in chronic asthma

Glucocorticoids are the prophylactic medication of choice for children with moderate-to-severe asthma that is occurring more frequently than once a week and is not controllable by bronchodilators used two or three times a week and sodium cromoglycate prophylaxis for 6–8 weeks (Warner, 1992). Inhaled glucocorticoid therapy with doses of beclomethasone or BUD of 400–600 µg per day divided into two or three doses showed no evidence of growth retardation in long-term studies and only minimal depression of endogenous cortisol secretion. Large-volume spacers, mouth-washing and discarding the fluid reduce systemic side-effects, as otherwise 90% of the aerosol is deposited in the oropharynx, swallowed and absorbed by the gastrointestinal tract. The optimal device depends on the child's age, as nebulizers or valved spacers with a face mask (up to 2 years), metered dose inhalers plus valved spacers (2–4 years), powder inhalers (5–8 years) and metered dose inhalers (older children) are available. If necessary, the dose can be increased to 2000 µg per day using a large-volume spacer. Oral or intravenous glucocorticoids (1–2 mg/kg per day prednisolone) should only be used in most severe cases that cannot be managed by maximal inhalative doses given four times a day and additional bronchodilators. Aerosol glucocorticoids should always be continued for their systemic steroid-sparing effects. Fluticasone propionate, a relatively new steroid, is supposed to have lower oral bio-availability and thus fewer systemic side-effects (Wolthers and Pedersen, 1993). Long-lasting steroids such as dexamethasone should be avoided.

Atopic eczema

Growth retardation as a complication of allergic childhood disease in general was described by Cohen et al (1940). The first definite dose-dependent, growth-suppressing effect of synthetic glucocorticoid treatment was reported in an eczematous child in 1956 (Blodgett et al, 1956). However, it took nearly half a century until the first paper about the growth pattern in children with atopic eczema appeared (Kristmundsdottir and David, 1987).

In this uncontrolled cross-sectional study, growth impairment was associated in particular with widespread eczema, the co-existence of asthma and the use of potent topical glucocorticoids. Height was below the 3rd percentile in 10% of the study population. When corrected for mid-parental height, this percentage increased to 22%. Interestingly, a disproportionate growth was found, with significantly reduced sitting height but normal subischial leg length. Skeletal maturation was likewise delayed in boys and girls, independent of the severity of dermatitis. Both findings are indicative of a postponed puberty. However, delayed sexual maturation has not yet been formally demonstrated as there are no longitudinal data available.

Subsequent papers have confirmed these first observations. Significant differences in height SDS were also shown between eczematous children without any history of asthma, anti-asthmatic medication or oral steroid therapy and healthy controls after correction for differences in age and parental height (Pike et al, 1989). Mean height SDS was found to be normal in pre-pubertal children with less than 50% of their skin surface area affected, whereas those with more than 50% of their skin affected were significantly shorter when compared both to the less severely diseased and to their own parental target height (Massarano et al, 1993). Regression analysis revealed only minor additional growth-retarding effects from topical steroid therapy and no effect from exclusion diets. Furthermore, normal weight and skinfold thickness in children with eczema made a nutritional aetiology of growth deterioration unlikely.

Fortunately, in most cases of eczema systemic glucocorticoid therapy can be avoided in favour of topical steroids. These should be used intermittently and early enough to ameliorate episodes of acute exacerbation. It has been suggested that permanent growth stunting may occur in children whose short stature is caused by long-term steroid therapy or whose severe eczema persists into adult life. If the short stature is attributed to severe disease alone, and if the disease remits before puberty, catch-up growth and attainment of full adult height is more likely (David, 1989).

Juvenile chronic arthritis

Influence of continuous versus intermittent glucocorticoid therapy on growth

Chronic inflammatory disease of the joints with childhood onset is usually referred to as juvenile chronic arthritis (JCA) in Europe and juvenile rheumatoid arthritis (JRA) in the USA. Glucocorticoid therapy is frequently needed when non-steroidal drugs fail to control symptoms, during acute episodes of deterioration and in the systemic form of JCA. Thus, it is generally extremely difficult to distinguish between the relative contributions of the illness itself and the secondary side-effects of medication when assessing growth disturbance in these children. Malnutrition, immobilization and precocious closure of epiphyseal growth plates inhibit growth independently of any therapy.

Besides the dose and duration of glucocorticoid therapy, the regimen of administration and the pharmacology of the drug are crucially important. In this respect, rheumatic children with three different treatment schedules were studied in a single centre investigation ($N = 36$) (Byron et al, 1983). Those receiving daily glucocorticoid therapy (0.6 mg prednisone/kg per day) ($N = 6$) all had a height velocity below the 3rd percentile after 1 year of follow-up, whereas 11 out of 13 patients on an alternate-day regimen (1 mg prednisone/kg on alternate days) were growing satisfactorily (Figure 2). A third group of children, switched from daily to intermittent therapy ($N = 17$), did not show a uniform growth pattern. Some of them, however, who failed to grow on daily dosages as low as 0.4 mg prednisone/kg body weight per day, started to gain height on 1 mg/kg body weight per day on alternate days. The same study demonstrated that mean resting cortisol levels, taken before awakening in the morning, correlated positively with height velocity after 1 year in each treatment group. All children who grew despite a still-suppressed hypothalamic–pituitary–adrenal axis, as assessed by insulin-induced hypoglycaemia, had been switched to alternate therapy.

The pharmacology of the specific glucocorticoid also determines the degree of growth retardation. Potency, in conjunction with the half-life of the compounds, is of major importance (plasma half-lives of cortisone/cortisol are 8–12 hours; prednisone/prednisolone and methylprednisolone, 12–36 hours; and dexamethasone and betamethasone, 36–72 hours). Levels of normal endogenously secreted cortisol are in the range of 32 µmol approximately equal to 12–13 mg/m^2 body surface area per day (see Chapter 4 in this volume). Dosages of about 45 mg/m^2 per day cortisol have

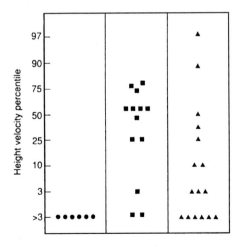

Figure 2. Comparison of daily (0.6 mg/kg) (●) and alternate-day (1 mg/kg) (■) prednisone therapy in juvenile chronic arthritis, for 1 year. (▲) Switched from daily to alternate-day prednisone. Reproduced from Byron et al (1983, *Journal of the Royal Society of Medicine* **76**: 452–457) with permission.

been shown to decrease growth rate and skeletal maturation in children without endocrine abnormalities (Blodgett et al, 1956). However, there is considerable interindividual variability in the appearance of steroid-induced side-effects. Hence it is difficult to define a dose of glucocorticoids that can be safely administered. Topical and intra-articular steroids, as used in patients with pauci- or monoarticular arthritis, particularly of the knee, do not generally interfere with statural growth (Falcini et al, 1991).

Short children with JCA generally show normal serum GH levels, but glucocorticoid treatment may lead to suppressed GH secretion. Therapy with exogenous GH (7.5–24 IU/m^2 per week) resulted in a significant increase of height velocity during the first year of treatment without an apparent effect on disease activity. Children with milder, oligoarticular forms and higher doses responded better than did those with systemic JCA and lower GH dosages (Butenandt, 1979; Davies et al, 1994). Long-term clinical trials of reasonable size are needed to draw more reliable conclusions on GH therapy in JCA.

Catch-up growth, even though often incomplete, can be expected after discontinuation or marked reduction of corticosteroids. However, because of irreversible alterations of growth plate cartilage and bone matrix as a consequence of the underlying disease and long-term glucocorticoid therapy, the longer the treatment period and the more it is extended into puberty, the less likely catch-up growth is to occur.

Guidelines for minimizing growth-depressing side-effects of glucocorticoids in JCA

The aim of treatment in more severe cases of JCA is not to suppress all symptoms and signs, but to reduce fever and pain and improve joint function and well-being, so that the child's social life is not unduly restricted. Daily divided dosages of oral glucocorticoids should be avoided. If the disease cannot be sufficiently controlled by non-steroidal therapy, the smallest possible dosage of glucocorticoids (up to 2 mg/kg body weight per day) should be given in a single morning dose on alternate days. If required, small, single, morning doses have to be added on the other days. Mono- and pauciarticular arthritis, in particular of the knee, should be considered for local therapy via intra-articular injection.

Clinical re-evaluation, aiming to reduce the steroid dosage in relation to the disease activity, is important. Although the individual sensitivity for glucocorticoids varies widely, doses above approximately 2 mg prednisolone equivalent per kg body weight on intermittent, or above 0.5 mg/kg body weight on daily, maintenance therapy are likely to suppress growth if given for a longer period.

In severe cases, non-steroidal immunosuppressive and cytostatic agents, details of which will not be reviewed here, can help to reduce the dose of glucocorticoids. GH treatment may be beneficial in certain children. Since this therapy is still experimental and an effect of GH on disease activity cannot be excluded by the present data, patients should be treated only in clinical studies. Adjunctive measures may include erythropoietin therapy, pain management and improvement of nutrition. Regular assessment of growth should be an integral part of any long-term corticosteroid therapy.

Inflammatory bowel disease

Growth failure frequently complicates the clinical course of inflammatory bowel disease in children. Absolute height deficits are reported in 10–40% of these patients (Motil and Grand, 1985), and height velocities may be reduced in 88%. This early growth retardation has been associated with permanent linear stunting in 17% of patients (Kirschner, 1990). The majority of children with growth delay have Crohn's disease rather than ulcerative colitis.

Growth failure in these children has been attributed to nutritional, hormonal and disease-related factors. Current evidence does not support primary hormonal disturbances as a cause of growth failure. Basal and stimulated serum GH levels are within the normal range. Low IGF-I levels in some patients with inflammatory bowel disease that paralleled their growth rates are most probably explained by concomitant malnutrition (Kirschner and Sutton, 1986). Indeed, malnutrition contributes significantly to growth failure, because growth resumes when children receive nutritional rehabilitation. In addition, nutritional therapy, alone or in conjunction with steroid therapy, reduces disease activity and enables a resumption of growth (Sanderson et al, 1987). Although the growth-depressing effects of glucocorticoids are well established, 60% of patients show linear growth delays before therapy is begun, whereas 80% show a reversal of growth failure after treatment is initiated (Berger et al, 1975). These observations suggest that the inflammatory process itself, rather than steroid usage *per se*, adversely affects growth. Motil et al (1993) tried to investigate the role of disease activity versus glucocorticoid therapy on growth failure in inflammatory bowel disease in a large prospective study. At least 23% of children showed evidence of growth failure. Growth deficits were equally prevalent regardless of the stage of pubertal development. Despite progressive sexual maturation, a delay in linear growth persisted throughout puberty. Significantly, the use of steroid therapy was not associated with linear growth delays, although high doses and long duration of usage tended to affect linear growth adversely. The authors concluded that the inflammatory process, rather than steroid use, has a predominant influence on the development of growth faltering. However, children in this study who received steroid therapy had clinical and biochemical evidence of more persistent inflammation. Hence, the inflammatory process itself may confound interpretations of the effects of steroid usage on the development of growth failure in inflammatory bowel disease. Taking these findings together, the suppression of disease activity appears to be the most important prerequisite for normal growth in inflammatory bowel disease. However, high doses of glucocorticoids over long periods of time should be avoided, because they certainly increase the risk of growth failure.

Nephrotic syndrome

Before the introduction of glucocorticoid therapy, uncontrolled nephrotic syndrome was associated with marked growth retardation. The main mechanisms involved were protein–calorie malnutrition secondary to poor appetite, protein loss in the urine and malabsorption due to oedema of the gastrointestinal tract. The growth-retarding effects of glucocorticoids in these patients soon became apparent. Patients who received repeated courses of high-dose steroids or prolonged maintenance therapy are at greatest risk of growth failure; an alternate-day schedule of steroid adminis-tration reduced growth velocity less than did daily administration. The key question is whether repetitive high-dose glucocorticoid treatment in this disorder only transiently retards growth velocity or definitely reduces final adult height. Between 5 and 24 years after their diagnosis, Foote et al (1985) examined the heights of 80 patients with steroid-responsive nephrotic syndrome who had received repeated courses of high-dose gluco-corticoids and prolonged maintenance therapy. Although at the time of taking glucocorticoids growth was suppressed, those who had completed growth had a mean height SDS of −0.22, equivalent to a height on the 40th percentile or 1.5 cm below average height, showing that standard gluco-corticoid therapy in steroid-responsive nephrotic syndrome does not systematically decrease ultimate height attainment. Total corticosteroid dose prescribed correlated only weakly with height SDS (Figure 3). There was no correlation between total dose of glucocorticoids and height when the post-pubertal patients were studied separately, indicating that their final height attainment was not affected significantly. A slight catch-up growth was observed in 33 patients who had been off treatment for at least 5 years.

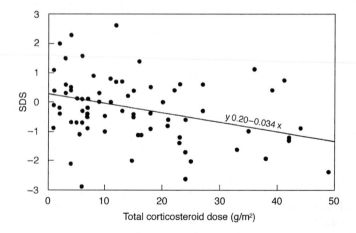

Figure 3. Height SDS versus total prednisolone dose in 72 patients with steroid-responsive nephrotic syndrome. Patients who had received large total doses of corticosteroids tended to be smaller than those who had received lower doses ($r = 0.38$, $P = 0.001$). Reproduced from Foote et al (1985, *Lancet* **ii:** 917–919, © The Lancet) with permission.

Polito et al (1986) studied the effects of alternate-day prednisone therapy for at least 1 year on statural growth over 1–6.5 years in 20 pre-pubertal children with frequently relapsing or steroid-dependent nephrotic syndrome. During the follow-up, 12 children showed variations in height SDS below 0.5, 7 gained more than 0.5 SDS, and 1 lost 0.5 SDS. This study supports the impression that glucocorticoid therapy in the nephrotic syndrome only rarely affects normal statural growth.

The situation might be different in patients who received long-term glucocorticoid therapy through adolescence. Rees et al (1988a) studied longitudinal height data and physical development in 29 boys and 12 girls taking long-term, alternate-day steroid treatment for steroid-sensitive nephrotic syndrome. Relative height worsened significantly only after the age of 10 years in relation to the duration of treatment, and was associated with a delay in the appearance of secondary sexual characteristics. Final height data in these children were not, however, reported. Hence the question remains of whether steroids only interfere with the onset and progression of puberty and the pubertal growth spurt, or whether adult height is negatively affected. If in individual cases unacceptable steroid side-effects and growth failure occur, induction of a prolonged relapse-free period with cyclophosphamide (Padilla and Brem, 1989) or cyclosporin A assures normal growth in most of the patients.

Renal transplantation

A well-functioning transplant in a child should theoretically restore the physiological conditions required for normal growth. However, growth rates after renal transplantation are highly variable and rarely fulfil the expectations of true catch-up growth. The main contributing factors to growth depression in children with renal transplants are glucocorticoid treatment for immunosuppression and reduced graft function. In addition, the growth response after a successful renal transplant depends on the age of the child and the severity of the growth failure at time of transplantation.

The cumulative amount of glucocorticoid is certainly a determinant of the growth rates achieved post-transplantation. The introduction of cyclosporin A for paediatric transplant patients in 1984 allowed a dose reduction of the concomitant glucocorticoid medication; however, improved growth rates were reported by only some investigators and not others (for a review, see Tönshoff and Mehls, 1994). Also, final height appears not to have been consistently improved by the introduction of cyclosporin A, in comparison with conventional immunosuppression.

The mode of administration of glucocorticoids appears to be related to their growth-depressing properties, an alternate-day regimen being more favourable than a daily dose. Broyer et al (1992) reported the first prospective controlled study involving 35 patients post-transplantation with a graft function of over 50 ml/min per 1.73 m² treated with either daily prednisone 0.25 mg/kg per day or an alternate-day regimen with the same cumulative steroid dosage. In pre-pubertal children on alternate-day therapy, a marked increase in height SDS of $+0.60 \pm 0.31$ SD during the first treatment year was observed when compared with pre-pubertal children on daily treatment (change in SDS per year 0.04 ± 0.31 SD). No acute rejection episode occurred in the alternate-day group. These data indicate that, at least in children with normal graft function, catch-up growth does occur during an alternate-day steroid regimen.

Only a few centres have studied the effect of glucocorticoid withdrawal on growth and graft function. Klare et al (1991) observed in a selected group of patients with stable graft function a mean increase in relative height of 0.8 ± 0.3 SD in the first year and 0.3 ± 0.2 SD in the second year after renal transplantation in 12 children with a serum creatinine level below 2.0 mg/dl. These data indicate that, at least in children with only slightly reduced graft function, cessation of glucocorticoids can induce catch-up growth. However, this regimen certainly increases the risk of graft rejection, with a reported incidence of 50–60% (Reisman et al, 1990). To reduce the risk of graft rejection, the patient has to be maintained on higher doses of cyclosporin, which, on the other hand, increase the risk of cyclosporin nephrotoxicity.

The age of the recipient at the time of transplantation also appears to influence the degree of growth improvement. In the experience of Ingelfinger et al (1981), only children below the age of 7 years demonstrated true catch-up growth after transplantation. Bosque et al (1983) reported better growth rates in patients with a bone age below 12 years at the time of transplantation. The importance of age-related changes in growth post-transplantation has recently been emphasized by Tejani et al (1993) with data from the North American Paediatric Renal Transplant Cooperative (NAPRTC) study. Catch-up growth (defined as a gain of relative height of at least 1 standard deviation in 2 years) occurred in 50% of the neonate to 1-year-old, 25% of the 2–5-year-old, 16% of the 6–12-year-old and 6% of the 13–17-year-old group. The authors drew the gloomy conclusion that growth outcome in children after transplantation has not substantially changed over the past decade.

Another determinant of normal growth post-transplant is the function of the renal graft. In the recent report from the NAPRTC Study following 300 children with a graft functioning for over 2 years, an increase in the serum creatinine level of 1.0 mg/dl was associated with a decrease in relative height of 0.15 SD years (Tejani et al, 1993). However, it is difficult to assess the impact of glomerular filtration rate on growth independently, because patients with poor graft function usually receive also higher amounts of glucocorticoid to suppress chronic graft rejection.

THIRD-GENERATION GLUCOCORTICOIDS: DEFLAZACORT

Deflazacort, an oxazoline derivative of prednisolone, was synthesized in 1967 (Nathanson et al, 1967). Since cortisone became available as the first exogenous glucocorticoid and subsequent hydrocortisone analogues were synthesized, this new heterocyclic glucocorticoid is referred to as a 'third-generation glucocorticoid'. Clinical studies suggest that deflazacort has fewer side-effects, while maintaining equipotent anti-inflammatory and immunosuppressive activity. In particular, a bone-sparing effect compared with prednisone and less interference with water, electrolyte, lipid and glucose metabolism have been reported. Data from experimental animals indicated that glycolytic enzyme activity and carbohydrate metabolism, which are of crucial importance for growth and mineralization of the epiphyseal cartilage, are better preserved with deflazacort than with prednisone (Kunin and Meyer, 1969: Russel et al, 1985). In vitro experiments, incubating bone or cartilage cells with different corticosteroids, supplement these findings. Deflazacort exhibits a lesser inhibitory effect on DNA synthesis, cell proliferation and collagen secretion in comparison with dexamethasone and methylprednisolone (Guenther et al, 1984; Kasperk et al, 1995). For a critical evaluation of deflazacort, it should be noted that there is no 'gold standard' available to compare equivalent immunosuppressive properties of different glucocorticoids. The present recommendation to substitute 1.2 mg deflazacort for 1 mg prednisone is based on short-term clinical studies on disease activity and animal experiments on the involution of lymphatic tissue and the reduction of lymphocyte subsets. These empirical data may not allow a valid comparison of biological activity in all circumstances.

The first report on the effects of deflazacort in children evaluated nine patients, aged 4–15 years (Balsan et al, 1987). In this heterogeneous study population on maintenance therapy for various renal diseases, immunoproliferative and connective tissue disorders, deflazacort was substituted for prednisone (1.2 mg/kg deflazacort for 1 mg/kg prednisone). Over a follow-up period of 10–16 months, symptom control was equally effective with deflazacort, while statural growth proceeded normally as before in all children, with a modest acceleration of growth velocity in some of them. Other steroid side-effects, including cushingoid appearance, hirsutism, striae and osteoporosis, which were initially present in most of these children, significantly improved.

Ferraris (Ferraris et al, 1992; Ferraris and Pasqualini, 1993) studied linear growth and GH secretion in children 4 years after renal transplantation who were substituted with deflazacort for methylprednisolone (mean maintenance dose of 0.3 for 0.2 mg/kg per day, assuming an equivalence of 1 mg prednisone to 0.8 mg methylprednisolone). Growth velocity in the pre-pubertal age group (9 children, Tanner stage 1) increased from 1.5 ± 0.3 to 3.2 ± 0.5 cm per year in the first, and to 4.1 ± 0.8 cm per year in the second, year of deflazacort treatment (8 of 9 children in Tanner stage 1). Bone age advanced by only 7 ± 6 months during the first 15 months after changing the treatment. This improved height velocity correlated with a higher mean spontaneous nocturnal GH secretion, which increased from 2.7 ± 0.5 to 4.3 ± 1.0 ng/ml during deflazacort medication. Also, the number of children responding with a GH peak of over 8 ng/ml to the arginine provocative test increased from 4 patients taking methylprednisolone to 8 out of 9 patients after replacement with deflazacort. Serum IGF-I levels remained unchanged after the shift in therapy. A decrease in cushingoid appearance, associated with a significant fall of the weight-to-height ratio was observed, especially during the first year of treatment, but returned to base-line levels in some of the patients during the second year. There was no evidence for adverse effects of deflazacort on graft function over the 2 years of follow-up.

Recently, the efficacy and side-effects of deflazacort versus prednisone in the treatment of idiopathic nephrotic syndrome were compared in a large randomized controlled study (Broyer et al, 1995a). Deflazacort allowed a better control of the idiopathic nephrotic syndrome with fewer relapses, but was associated with similar side-effects in terms of growth velocity, with a tendency to be less deleterious on bone density.

Preliminary experience with deflazacort in children with JCA gives less clear evidence for the supposed growth-preserving effect of deflazacort. A randomized, double-blind trial of this drug versus prednisone (assuming an equivalence of 5 to 6 for prednisone to deflazacort; $N = 7$ per group) failed to show a significantly better height gain in pre-pubertal children after 1 year of observation (Loftus et al, 1991). Relative spinal bone mineral density for height and weight, however, was better maintained in the deflazacort group.

Taken together, there is an increasing body of evidence for a favourable influence of deflazacort on glucocorticoid-induced side-effects, for example cushingoid appearance and especially osteoporosis. However, since under clinical conditions the dosage of deflazacort equivalent to that of prednisone is incompletely defined, the fewer side-effects of deflazacort may also be due to a slight reduction of the equivalent glucocorticoid dosage. The possible role of deflazacort in preserving childhood growth potential also needs further evaluation. Long-term observations and larger well-controlled and comparative studies are required to assess whether better short-term growth during deflazacort treatment will lead to an improvement in final height attainment.

CONCOMITANT TREATMENT WITH GLUCOCORTICOIDS AND GH/IGF-I

Reversal of the catabolic effects of glucocorticoids

Two rationales for GH therapy of glucocorticoid-induced growth failure and catabolism can be given: (1) in those individuals who secrete abnormal amounts of GH, rhGH treatment can be considered as substitution therapy, and (2) in those children who secrete normal amounts of GH but have decreased biologically available IGF, rhGH is able to restore IGF bio-activity (Tönshoff et al, 1993).

Previously, the prevailing view was that it would be difficult to counteract the growth-inhibiting effects of glucocorticoids by con-comitant treatment with GH or IGF-I, because the inhibitory effects of glucocorticoids appeared to be operative mainly at the tissue level. The first clinical studies on the effect of GH on glucocorticoid-induced growth failure gave inconclusive results. Morris et al (1968) observed no significant metabolic response to exogenous human GH in glucocorticoid-treated children, and only minimal nitrogen retention in nitrogen balance studies. In the same study, prolonged GH therapy with large doses given for periods of 4–8 months to six glucocorticoid-treated children did not stimulate longitudinal growth. The same negative result of GH therapy was observed in growth-retarded children with inflammatory bowel disease (McCaffery et al, 1974). In contrast, Butenandt (1979) reported positive short-term effects of GH therapy in growth-retarded children with rheumatoid arthritis. Recently, Allen and Goldberg (1992) studied the effects of GH treatment, 0.3 mg/kg per week for 6–21 months, in seven slowly growing children with various diseases treated with glucocorticoids. Mean height velocity increased from 3.4 ± 0.7 cm per year to 6.7 ± 0.8 cm per year. These conflicting results are probably explained by the small numbers of patients studied, short treatment periods, inclusion of pubertal patients, variations in the activity of the underlying disease and infrequent administration as well as discontinuation of GH therapy.

Since the recent availability of rhGH in virtually unlimited amounts, there is growing scientific interest in a possible beneficial effect of GH and/or IGF-I on glucocorticoid-induced growth failure and catabolism. Kovacs et al (1991) demonstrated that methylprednisolone inhibited weight and length gain in rats in a dose-dependent manner, and that rhGH was able to compensate for the growth-depressing effects of methylprednisolone. The same beneficial effects of rhGH were observed in uraemic rats, in which glucocorticoids completely inhibited growth. Horber and Haymond (1990) demonstrated that rhGH was able to prevent the protein catabolic side-effects of prednisone in 32 healthy adult volunteers. Prednisone 0.8 mg/kg per day for 7 days induced protein wasting, whereas rhGH 0.1 mg/kg per day resulted in a positive protein balance, calculated from leucine kinetic data or nitrogen balance values. When GH was added to prednisone therapy, the glucocorticoid-induced protein catabolism was prevented. Bennet and Haymond (1992) extended these studies by showing that the anabolic effects were observed in subjects receiving long-term treatment with one quarter of the dose of glucocorticoids and one eighth of the dose of GH. Based on leucine kinetic data, negative protein balance during prednisone treatment was due to increased proteolysis, whereas GH had no effect on proteolysis, but increased whole body protein synthesis. As prednisone and GH had differential effects on fuel metabolism and insulin antagonism, the authors assumed in part independent mechanisms in which GH and prednisone may reciprocally regulate the oxidation of protein and fat while decreasing the efficiency of glucose disposal. These data suggest that some of the catabolic effects of glucocorticoids on protein can indeed be countered by human GH. However, these benefits were obtained at the cost of markedly increased concentrations of circulating insulin and glucose, indicating increased insulin resistance.

Mauras and Beaufrere (1995) examined the question of whether similar anabolic effects can be obtained by rhIGF-I in the prednisone-treated subjects without a reduction in carbohydrate tolerance. In this study, IGF-I treatment abolished the increase in proteolysis and markedly reduced the increase in leucine oxidation in prednisone-treated subjects. Furthermore, unlike in the GH-treated subjects, the amelioration of steroid-induced protein catabolism was seen with no rise in plasma glucose and with a significant reduction in circulating insulin levels.

GH treatment in children post-kidney transplantation

Persistent growth failure after renal transplantation is mainly due to reduced graft function and concomitant glucocorticoid medication. If catch-up growth cannot be achieved by an alternate-day steroid regimen, and discontinuation of glucocorticoids appears as an intolerable risk for graft survival, rhGH therapy may be initiated. However, not all safety aspects of rhGH therapy for this group of children have been sufficiently studied (see below).

Efficacy of GH treatment

The short-term growth response to rhGH has been documented in a number of open-labelled prospective studies with observation periods of 1 year, 2 years (for a review, see Tönshoff and Fine, 1995) and 3 years (Tönshoff et al, 1993). Height velocity in the first treatment year in pre-pubertal children can clearly be doubled by rhGH treatment. The growth-promoting effect of rhGH moderately declines in the second and third treatment years, as observed in GH trials for other treatment indications. However, because the natural course of growth in children post-transplantation is frequently one of progressive growth deceleration, even modest improvement of growth rates, if sustained, can result in normalization of longitudinal growth. In our experience, the short-term growth response to rhGH was not significantly correlated with the dose of prednisolone administered (range 2.3–9.1 mg/m^2 per day), graft function as estimated by creatinine clearances (range 19–88 ml/min per 1.73 m^2), the degree of stunting at base-line, base-line height velocity and chronological age. However, a relatively tight inverse correlation was found between the growth response to rhGH and the degree of bone age delay (Figure 4) (Tönshoff et al, 1996). Hence, the degree of bone age delay appears to be a helpful clinical predictor of the response to rhGH in short pre-pubertal children post-renal transplantation.

Promising preliminary results have also been obtained in growth-retarded pubertal children post-transplantation: 18 adolescents demonstrated an impressive growth response to rhGH, with a mean increment in height after 2 years of rhGH therapy of 15.7 ± 5.1 cm, compared with 5.8 ± 3.4 cm in retrospectively matched control individuals (Hokken-Koelega et al, 1994). This growth response occurred independently whether 4 or 8 IU rhGH/m^2 per day were given.

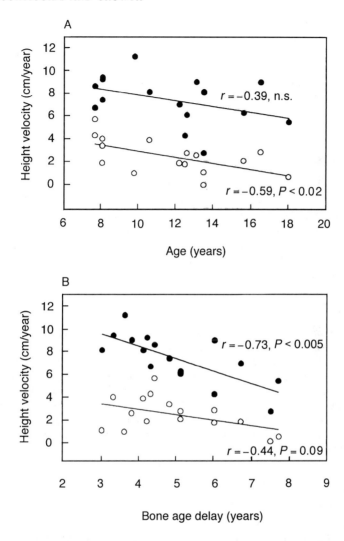

Figure 4. (A) Base-line height velocity (○) and height velocity after 1 year of rhGH (●) as a function of chronological age. There was a significant inverse correlation between base-line height velocity and chronological age ($r = -0.59$, $P < 0.02$). (B) Base-line height velocity (○) and height velocity after 1 year of rhGH (●) as a function of bone age delay. There was a significant inverse correlation between height velocity after 1 year of rhGH and the degree of bone age delay ($r = -0.73$, $P < 0.005$). Reproduced from Tönshoff et al (in press, *British Journal of Clinical Practice*) with permission.

Safety of GH treatment

Assessment of the risks of GH treatment in children undergoing renal allografts naturally focuses on any deleterious effect on the survival of the transplant. There are theoretical reasons for the concern that the immunostimulatory effects of GH in children might reduce the effectiveness of the immunosuppression by glucocorticoids (Hokken-Koelega et al, 1994). Indeed, there is some evidence from a preliminary analysis of a randomized prospective study that GH might slightly increase the rejection rate in high-risk patients who already experienced multiple rejection episodes before initiation of GH therapy, but not in those with no or only 1 rejection episode (Broyer et al, 1995b). More research is needed to assess this risk more accurately and perhaps to define more clearly the patient population likely to benefit from GH treatment.

The main metabolic change induced by exogenous GH in our experience (Tönshoff et al, 1993) was an increase in insulin secretion, which continued to progress during the 3 years of treatment, whereas glucose tolerance, as measured by an oral glucose tolerance test and the determination of glycosylated haemoglobin concentrations, did not change in any of the studied children. Hyperinsulinaemia and relative insulin resistance are well-known general effects of exogenous GH administration. Especially in children with renal allografts, this metabolic change may be potentially harmful, since a pre-existing relative insulin resistance, from the combined effect of pharmacological doses of glucocorticoids and uraemia, seems to be further aggravated by rhGH therapy. The long-term consequences of increased insulin secretion are uncertain, but hyperinsulinaemia per se has been implicated as a direct causative factor in the pathogenesis of atherosclerosis (Stout, 1979). In addition, chronic stimulation of the pancreatic β-cells by GH treatment may lead to exhaustion of insulin secretory capacity over time, as observed in patients with acromegaly. However, at least in short normal children treated with a very high dose of GH (55 IU/m^2 per week), the hyperinsulinaemia and relative insulin resistance observed after 2 years of rhGH administration were reversible after GH therapy was discontinued (Lesage et al, 1991), indicating that these alterations in insulin sensitivity are only transient. Nevertheless, it is recommended that, while receiving combined treatment with glucocorticoids and rhGH, children should be closely monitored for disturbances in glucose metabolism.

SUMMARY

Growth failure is a frequent side effect of long-term, high-dose glucocorticoid therapy in children. Pharmacological doses of glucocorticoids interfere at different levels with the integrity of the somatotrophic hormone axis. The majority of patients on chronic corticosteroid medication demonstrate overt GH hyposecretion, apparently due to enhancement of hypothalamic somatostatin release. Glucocorticoids also inhibit IGF bioactivity by the induction of IGF inhibitors, and stimulate the production of certain IGFBPs. In addition, glucocorticoids inhibit growth directly at the tissue level by suppression of local growth factors and of skeletal tissue matrix production. If systemic application is necessary, optimization of glucocorticoid therapy in chronic paediatric diseases preferably comprises low-dose, alternate-day treatment. Topical application whenever possible, as in atopic eczema and monoarticular JCA, is preferable. Likewise, inhalational glucocorticoid therapy in bronchial asthma clearly reduces the risk of growth failure in these children and may be associated with a normal height prognosis. In children post-renal transplantation, concomitant treatment with cyclosporin A for immunosuppression allows low-dose glucocorticoid medication, which, in particular as alternate-day therapy, improves growth in some but not all children. The new glucocorticoid deflazacort appears to have fewer side-effects with respect to steroid-induced osteopenia and cushingoid appearance; a beneficial effect on longitudinal growth is not clearly established. Recent experimental and clinical data indicate that the catabolic and growth-depressing effects of glucocorticoids can be counterbalanced by concomitant anabolic treatment with rhGH. The potential role of rhIGF-I is less well investigated. Treatment with rhGH is able to antagonize several side-effects of long-term glucocorticoid administration, such as growth failure, protein wasting and osteoporosis. However, rhGH therapy in this setting must still be considered experimental, since a possible interference of rhGH with the immunosuppressive action of glucocorticoids is not excluded, in particular in children after organ transplantation.

REFERENCES

Aitman TJ, Palmer RG, Loftus J et al (1989) Serum IGF-I levels and growth failure in juvenile chronic arthritis. *Clinical and Experimental Rheumatology* **7:** 557–561.

Allen DB & Goldberg BD (1992) Stimulation of collagen synthesis and linear growth by growth hormone in glucocorticoid-treated children. *Pediatrics* **89:** 416–421.

Allen DB, Mullen ML & Mullen B (1994) A meta-analysis of the effect of oral and inhaled corticosteroids on growth. *Allergy and Clinical Immunology* **93:** 967–976.

Balfour-Lynn L (1986) Growth and childhood asthma. *Archives of Disease in Childhood* **61:** 1049–1055.

Balsan S, Steru D, Bourdeau A et al (1987) Effects of long-term maintenance therapy with a new glucocorticoid, deflazacort, on mineral metabolism and statural growth. *Calcified Tissue International* **40:** 303–309.

Bang P, Degerblad M, Thoren M et al (1993) Insulin-like growth factor (IGF) I and II and IGF binding protein (IGFBP) 1, 2 and 3 in serum from patients with Cushing's syndrome. *Acta Endocrinologica* **128:** 397–404.

Bennet WM & Haymond MW (1992) Growth hormone and lean tissue catabolism during long-term glucocorticoid treatment. *Clinical Endocrinology* **36:** 161–164.

Berger M, Gribetz D & Korelitz BI (1975) Growth retardation in children with ulcerative colitis: the effect of medical and surgical treatment. *Pediatrics* **55:** 459–467.

Blodgett FM, Burgin L, Iezzoni D et al (1956) Effects of prolonged cortisone therapy on the statural growth, skeletal maturation and metabolic status of children. *New England Journal of Medicine* **254:** 636–641.

Bosque M, Munian A, Bewick M et al (1983) Growth after renal transplants. *Archives of Disease in Childhood* **58:** 110–114.

Broyer M, Guest G & Gagnadoux M (1992) Growth rate in children receiving alternate-day corticosteroid treatment after kidney transplantation. *Journal of Pediatrics* **120:** 721–725.

Broyer M, Guest G, Crosnier H & Berard E, on the behalf of the French Society for Pediatric Nephrology (1995b). A multicentric open randomized controlled study of rhGH therapy in short children after kidney transplantation. *Journal of the American Society of Nephrology* **6:** 1075 (abstract).

Broyer M, Terzi F, Gagnadoux MF et al (1995a) A randomized double blind study of deflazacort (D) versus prednisone (P) in the treatment of idiopathic nephrotic syndrome (NS). *Journal of the American Society of Nephrology* **6:** 414 (abstract).

330
B. TÖNSHOFF ET AL

Butenandt O (1979) Rheumatoid arthritis and growth retardation in children: treatment with human growth hormone. *European Journal of Pediatrics* **130:** 15–28.

Byron MA, Jackson J & Ansell BM (1983) Effect of different corticosteroid regimes on hypothalamic–pituitary–adrenal axis and growth in juvenile chronic arthritis. *Journal of the Royal Society of Medicine* **76:** 452–457.

Casanueva FF, Burguera B & Tome M (1990) Depending on the time of administration, dexamethasone potentiates or blocks growth hormone-releasing hormone-induced growth hormone release in man. *Neuroendocrinology* **47:** 46–49.

Cohen MB & Abram LE (1948) Growth pattern of allergic children. *Journal of Allergy* **19:** 165–171.

Cohen MB, Weller RR & Cohen S (1940) Anthropometry in children. Progress in allergic children as shown by increments in height, weight and maturity. *American Journal of Diseases of Childhood* **60:** 1058–1066.

David TJ (1989) Short stature in children with atopic eczema. *Acta Dermato-venereologica* **144 (supplement):** 41–44.

Davies UM, Rooney M, Preece MA et al (1994) Treatment of growth retardation in juvenile chronic arthritis with recombinant human growth hormone. *Journal of Rheumatology* **21:** 153–158.

Elders MJ, Wingfield BS, McNatt ML et al (1975) Glucocorticoid therapy in children. Effect on somatomedin secretion. *American Journal of Disease in Childhood* **129:** 1393–1396.

Falcini F, Taccetti G, Trapani S et al (1991) Growth retardation in juvenile chronic arthritis patients treated with steroids. *Clinical and Experimental Rheumatology* **9 (supplement 6):** 37–40.

Falliers CJ, Tan LS & Szentivanyi J (1963) Childhood asthma and steroid therapy as influences on growth—how to interfere with a child's growth without really trying. *American Journal of Diseases of Children* **105:** 127–137.

Ferraris JR & Pasqualini T (1993) Therapy with a new glucocorticoid: effect of deflazacort on linear growth and growth hormone secretion in renal transplantation. *Journal of Rheumatology* **20 (supplement 37):** 43–46.

Ferraris JR, Day PF, Gutman R et al (1992) Effect of therapy with a new glucocorticoid, deflazacort, on linear growth and growth hormone secretion after renal transplantation. *Journal of Pediatrics* **121:** 809–813.

Foote KD, Brocklebank JT & Meadow SR (1985) Height attainment in children with steroid-responsive nephrotic syndrome. *Lancet* **ii:** 917–919.

Gabrielsson BG, Carmignac DF, Flavell DM & Robinson CAF (1995) Steroid regulation of growth hormone (GH) receptor and GH binding protein messenger ribonucleic acids in the rat. *Endocrinology* **133:** 2445–2452.

Giustina A, Bossoni S, Bodini C et al (1992) Arginine normalizes the growth hormone (GH) response to GH-releasing hormone in adult patients receiving chronic immunosuppressive daily glucocorticoid therapy. *Journal of Clinical Endocrinology and Metabolism* **74:** 1301–1305.

Green H, Morikawa M & Nixon T (1985) A dual effector theory of growth-hormone action. Models and hypotheses. *Differentiation* **29:** 195–198.

Green OC, Winter RF, Dawahara FS et al (1978) Pharmakokinetic studies of prednisolone in children: plasma levels, half-life values, and correlation with physiologic assays for growth and immunity. *Journal of Pediatrics* **93:** 299–303.

Guenther HL, Felix R & Fleisch H (1984) Comparative study of deflazacort, a new synthetic corticosteroid, and dexamethasone on the synthesis of collagen in different rat bone cell populations and rabbit articular chondrocytes. *Calcified Tissue International* **36:** 145–152.

Hokken-Koelega ACS, Stijnen T, De Ridder MAJ et al (1994) Growth hormone therapy in growth-retarded adolescents after renal transplantation. *Lancet* **343:** 1313–1317.

Hollman GA & Allen DB (1988) Overt glucocorticoid excess due to inhaled corticosteroid therapy. *Pediatrics* **81:** 452–455.

Horber FF & Haymond MW (1990) Human growth hormone prevents the protein catabolic side effects of prednisone in humans. *Journal of Clinical Investigation* **86:** 265–272.

Ingelfinger JR, Grupe WE, Harmon WB et al (1981) Growth acceleration following renal transplantation in children less than 7 years of age. *Pediatrics* **68:** 255–259.

Isaksson OPG, Lindahl A, Nilsson A & Isgaard J (1987) Mechanism of the stimulatory effect of growth hormone on longitudinal bone growth. *Endocrine Revue* **8(4):** 426–438.

Jux C, Leiber K, Hügel U et al (1996) Dexamethasone inhibits GH stimulated and IGF-I mediated proliferation by reduction of paracrine IGF-I secretion and somatotropic receptor down-regulation in cultured growth plate chondrocytes. *Tenth International Congress of Endocrinology*, San Francisco, (abstract) (in press).

Kasperk C, Schneider U, Sommer U et al (1995) Differential effects of glucocorticoids on human osteoblastic cell metabolism in vitro. *Calcified Tissue International* **57**: 120–126.

King APJ & Carter-Su C (1995) Dexamethasone-induced antagonism of growth hormone (GH) action by down-regulation of GH binding in 3T3-F442A fibroblasts. *Endocrinology* **136**: 4796–4803.

Krischner BS (1990) Growth and development in chronic inflammatory bowel disease. *Acta Paediatrica Scandinavica* **366 (supplement)**: 98–104.

Kirschner BS & Suton MM (1986) Somatomedin-C levels in growth impaired children and adolescents with chronic inflammatory bowel disease. *Gastroenterology* **91**: 830–836.

Klare B, Strom TM, Hahn H et al (1991) Remarkable long-term prognosis and excellent growth in kidney-transplant children under cyclosporine monotherapy. *Transplantation Proceedings* **23**: 1013–1017.

Klaus G, von Eichel B, May T et al (1994) Synergistic effects of parathyroid hormone and 1,25-dihydroxyvitamin D3 on proliferation and vitamin D receptor expression of rat growth cartilage cells. *Endocrinology* **135**: 1307–1315.

Kovacs G, Fine RN, Worgall S et al (1991) Growth hormone prevents steroid-induced growth depression in health and uremia. *Kidney International* **40**: 1032–1040.

Kristmundsdottir F & David TJ (1987) Growth impairment in children with atopic eczema. *Journal of the Royal Society of Medicine* **80**: 9–12.

Kunin AS & Meyer AS (1969) The effect of cortisone on the intermediary metabolism of epiphyseal cartilage of rats. *Archives of Biochemistry and Biophysics* **29**: 421–430.

Lesage C, Walker J, Landier F et al (1991) Near normalization of adolescent height with growth hormone therapy in very short children without growth hormone deficiency. *Journal of Pediatrics* **119**: 29–34.

Loftus J, Allen R, Hesp R et al (1991) Randomised, double-blind trial of deflazacort versus prednisolone in juvenile chronic (or rheumatoid) arthritis: a relatively bone-sparing effect of deflazacort. *Pediatrics* **88**: 428–436.

Luo J & Murphy LJ (1989) Dexamethasone inhibits growth hormone induction of insulin-like growth factor-I (IGF-I) messenger ribonucleic acid (mRNA) in hypophysectomized rats and reduces IGF-I mRNA abundance in the intact rat. *Endocrinology* **125**: 165–171.

McCaffery TD, Nasr K, Lawrence AM & Kirsner JB (1974) Effect of administered human growth hormone on growth retardation in inflammatory bowel disease. *Digestive Diseases* **19**: 411–416.

Massarano AA, Hollis S, Devlin J & David TJ (1993) Growth in atopic eczema. *Archives of Disease in Childhood* **68**: 677–679.

Mauras N & Beaufrere B (1995) rhIGF-I enhances whole body protein anabolism and significantly diminishes the protein-catabolic effects of prednisone in humans without a diabetogenic effect. *Journal of Clinical Endocrinology and Metabolism* **80**: 869–874.

Miell JP, Taylor AM, Jones J et al (1993) The effects of dexamethasone treatment on immunoreactive and bioactive insulin-like growth factor (IGFs) and IGF binding proteins in normal male volunteers. *Journal of Endocrinology* **23**: 45–49.

Morris HG, Jorgensen JR & Jenkins SA (1968) Plasma growth hormone concentration in corticosteroid-treated children. *Journal of Clinical Investigation* **47**: 427–435.

Motil KJ & Grand RJ (1985) Nutritional management of inflammatory bowel disease. *Pediatric Clinics of North America* **32**: 447–469.

Motil KJ, Grand RJ, Davis-Kraft L et al (1993) Growth failure in children with inflammatory bowel disease: a prospective study. *Gastroenterology* **105**: 681–691.

Nathanson G, Winters G & Testa E (1967) Steroids possessing nitrogen atoms. III. Synthesis of new highly active corticoids [17α, 16α-d] oxazoline steroids. *Journal of Medicinal Chemistry* **10**: 799–802.

Ninan TK & Russell G (1992) Asthma, inhaled corticosteroid treatment, and growth. *Archives of Disease in Childhood* **67**: 703–705.

Padilla R & Brem AS (1989) Linear growth of children with nephrotic syndrome: effect of alkylating agents. *Pediatrics* **84**: 495–499.

Pike MG, Chang CL, Atherton DJ et al (1989) Growth in atopic eczema: a controlled study by questionnaire. *Archives of Disease in Childhood* **64**: 1566–1569.

Polito C, Oporto MR, Totino SF et al (1986) Normal growth of nephrotic children during long-term alternate-day prednisone therapy. *Acta Paediatrica Scandinavica* **75**: 245–250.

Rees L, Greene SA, Adlard P et al (1988a) Growth and endocrine function in steroid sensitive nephrotic syndrome. *Archives of Disease in Childhood* **63**: 484–490.

Rees L, Greene SA, Adlard P et al (1988b) Growth and endocrine function after renal transplantation. *Archives of Disease in Childhood* **63**: 1326–1332.

Reisman L, Lieberman KV, Burrows L & Schanzer H (1990) Follow-up of cyclosporine-treated pediatric renal allograft recipients after cessation of prednisone. *Transplantation* **49**: 76–80.

Robinson ICAF, Gabrielsson B, Klaus G et al (1995) Glucocorticoids and growth problems. *Acta Paediatrica* **411 (supplement)**: 81–86.

Russel JE, Gennari C, Imbimbo B & Avioli LV (1985) Effects of deflazacort and the L-6485 metabolite on epiphyseal cartilage carbohydrate metabolism: comparison with prednisone. *Hormone and Metabolism Research* **17**: 402–405.

Salter HH (1868) *On Asthma: its Pathology and Treatment*, 2nd edn. London: Churchill.

Sanderson IR, Udeen S, Davies PSW et al (1987) Remission induced by an elemental diet in small bowel Crohn's disease. *Archives of Disease in Childhood* **61**: 123–127.

Schaefer F, Hamill G, Stanhope R et al (1991) Pulsatile growth hormone secretion in prepubertal patients with chronic renal failure. *Journal of Pediatrics* **119**: 568–577.

Silbermann M & Maor G (1978) Mechanisms of glucocorticoid-induced growth retardation: impairment of cartilage mineralization. *Acta Anatomica* **101**: 140–149.

Slootweg MC, de Groot RP, Herrman-Erlee MP et al (1991) Growth hormone induces expression of c-jun and jun B oncogenes and employs a protein kinase C signal transduction pathway for the induction of c-fos oncogene expression. *Journal of Molecular Endocrinology* **6**: 179–188.

Stout RW (1979) Diabetes and atherosclerosis—the role of insulin. *Diabetologica* **16**: 141–145.

Tejani A, Fine RN, Alexander S et al (1993) Factors predictive of sustained growth in children after renal transplantation. *Journal of Pediatrics* **122**: 397–402.

Tönshoff B & Mehls O (1994) Use of rhGH posttransplantation in children. In Tejani AH & Fine RN (eds) *Pediatric Renal Transplantation*, pp 441–459. New York: Wiley-Liss.

Tönshoff B & Fine RN (1995) Growth and growth hormone treatment in children with renal insufficiency. In Nissenson AR, Fine RN & Gentile DE (eds) *Clinical Dialysis*, 3rd edn, pp 549–573. East Norwalk, CT: Appleton & Lange.

Tönshoff B, Haffner D, Mehls O et al (1993) Efficacy and safety of growth hormone treatment in short children with renal allografts: three year experience. *Kidney International* **44**: 199–207.

Tönshoff B, Haffner D, Albers N et al (1996) Predictors of growth response to growth hormone in short prepubertal children post renal transplantation. *British Journal of Clinical Practice* (in press).

Unterman TG & Phillips LS (1985) Glucocorticoid effects on somatomedins and somatomedin inhibitors. *Journal of Clinical Endocrinology and Metabolism* **61**: 618–626.

Veldhuis JD, Lizarralde G, Iranmanesh A (1992) Divergent effects of short term glucocorticoid excess on the gonadotropic and somatotropic axes in normal men. *Journal of Clinical Endocrinology and Metabolism* **74**: 96–102.

Warner JO (1992) Asthma: a follow up statement from an international paediatric asthma consensus group. *Archives of Disease in Childhood* **67**: 240–248.

Wehrenberg WB, Janowski BA, Piering AW et al (1990) Glucocorticoids: potent inhibitors and stimulators of growth hormone secretion. *Endocrinology* **126**: 3200–3203.

Wolthers OD & Pedersen S (1993) Short term growth during treatment with inhaled fluticasone propionate and beclomethasone dipropionate. *Archives of Disease in Childhood* **68**: 673–676.

7

The effect of chemotherapy on growth and endocrine function in childhood

HAMISH WALLACE
CHRISTOPHER J. H. KELNAR

The last three decades have witnessed a substantial and sustained improvement in survival from most forms of childhood cancer. The 5-year survival rate for childhood lymphoblastic leukaemia towards the end of the 1960s was around 10%, while today more than 65% of these children can now be cured. The number of long-term survivors from childhood cancer is now increasing exponentially such that it has been estimated that by the year 2000 at least 1 in 1000 young adults in their third decade will have been cured of childhood cancer.

The major challenge for this generation of children's cancer specialists is to sustain the significant improvement in survival rates while at the same time minimizing the treatment-induced late effects. Treatment of cancer in childhood may result in a variety of clinical presentations, including short stature, delayed or precocious puberty, hypothyroidism, thyroid tumours, infertility and varying degrees of hypopituitarism (Wallace, 1996). Radiotherapy has been a major source of late-effects morbidity, with cranial irradiation being clearly implicated in the development of growth retardation in the long-term survivors. The effect of cranial radiotherapy on the hypothalamic–pituitary axis is dose related, and the fractionation schedule is also important. Modern chemotherapy protocols for the management of childhood leukaemia aim to avoid cranial irradiation as CNS-directed therapy, and therefore the role of intensive chemotherapy on growth and endocrine function has assumed increasing importance.

Cytotoxic chemotherapy disrupts normal cell division in rapidly dividing cells; however, the cells that are involved with growth, such as the cells of the hypothalamic–pituitary axis, the liver and the growth plate, are not generally undergoing rapid cell division, which may make the effects of chemotherapy on the growth axis subtle.

GROWTH AND CHEMOTHERAPY

Acute lymphoblastic leukaemia (ALL)

There has been much controversy generated over the growth patterns and growth hormone (GH) requirements of children treated for ALL. The

Baillière's Clinical Paediatrics—
Vol. 4, No. 2, May 1996
ISBN 0–7020–2180–6
0963–6714/96/020333 + 15 $12.00/00

prevalence of GH deficiency in those children who receive cranial irradiation as CNS-directed treatment depends not only on the total dose received, but also on the number of fractions, the fraction size and the duration of the radiation schedule (Shalet et al, 1979). There is no doubt that the duration and nature of the combination cytotoxic chemotherapy received by children with ALL influences the growth prognosis. A study of 82 children treated for ALL with combination chemotherapy and cranial irradiation showed that in those children who received 2 years of chemotherapy, catch-up growth was seen in the third year after diagnosis, irrespective of the radiation schedule; when chemotherapy was given for a third year, this catch-up growth was delayed by a year (Clayton et al, 1988). An Australian study (Kirk et al, 1987) reported significant growth retardation after treatment for ALL with cranial irradiation and combination chemotherapy. At 4 years from diagnosis, 32% of the survivors had shown a decrease in standing height by more than 1 standard deviation from the population mean, while at 6 years from diagnosis, this figure had risen to 71%. These findings contrast with those of the British study (Clayton et al, 1988). In the British study, the mean standing height standard deviation score (SDS) 6 years after diagnosis was −0.44, compared with −1.5 in the Australian study (Figure 1). The cranial irradiation schedules received by the two groups of children were similar, and therefore the different degree of growth retardation in these two studies is unlikely to be explained by a variation in the prevalence of GH deficiency. There is no doubt that the chemotherapy protocol received by the Australian children (LSA_2L_2 protocol) is more 'intense', both in content and duration, than the British

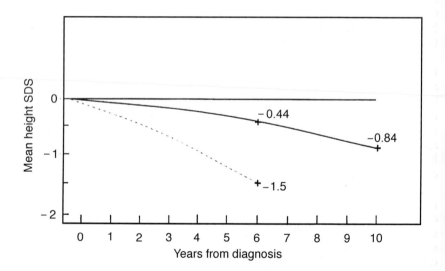

Figure 1. Growth retardation after treatment for ALL: comparison of two studies employing different chemotherapy protocols. (—) British study (Clayton et al, 1988); (---) Australian study (Kirk et al, 1987).

schedule, and we believe this is the major reason for the dissimilar growth pattern seen in the two studies.

Further support for the role of intensive chemotherapy on growth retardation comes from a study by Mohnike et al (1995) in which the effect of two different chemotherapy protocols for ALL was studied. The height SDS decreased significantly with increasing time from treatment in those children who received the more intensive chemotherapy protocol—the same protocol received by the Australian children (Kirk et al, 1987).

In a continuing longitudinal study of height and sitting height in 31 children on treatment for ALL, we have found a significant reduction in height SDS over the first 10 months of treatment followed by an improvement (Ahmed et al, personal communication). There is a further significant fall in height SDS at 13 months, which is followed by a sustained improvement. There was a suggestion that those children who received a third intensification block of treatment were more adversely affected, although this was not significant owing to small numbers.

A study by Moell et al (1994) in 179 girls treated for ALL in Scandinavia showed no difference in pre-pubertal growth between those girls who had received cranial irradiation and those who had not. Pubertal growth was, however, significantly worse in those girls who received cranial irradiation, as was the overall change in height SDS. In an earlier study of 13 girls who had received cranial irradiation (20–24 Gy), Moell et al (1988) showed that during a 24-hour GH profile, a pulsatile pattern of GH secretion was maintained, but the amplitude of the GH peaks was significantly reduced in comparison with normal controls. This loss of GH amplitude was more marked in the pubertal girls. More recently, low-dose cranial irradiation has been shown to cause subtle perturbations in GH secretion during puberty (Crowne et al, 1992). The intensity of the chemotherapy delivered to the Scandinavian girls was less than that currently administered (no intensification blocks), which may explain the normal pre-pubertal growth observed.

In an American study by Sklar et al (1993) of 127 children who had been treated for ALL, 38 children who did not receive cranial irradiation showed a significant reduction in height SDS score between diagnosis and final height (−0.49), although this height loss was less than for those who received cranial irradiation. By contrast, other workers have found no significant reduction in final height in children treated with chemotherapy alone (Katz et al, 1991; Hokken-Keolega et al, 1993; Holm et al, 1994; Moell et al, 1994). This is likely to reflect a difference in the intensity of chemotherapy protocols.

A retrospective study (Davies et al, 1994) of 142 long-term survivors of ALL showed that combination chemotherapy with either 18 or 24 Gy cranial irradiation as CNS-directed therapy may cause significant loss of standing height. More interestingly, at final height 82% had relatively shorter backs than legs, and in nearly one quarter of patients studied the disproportion was significant, with more than 2 SDs difference between sitting height and leg length. None of the patients had received spinal irradiation. This study also showed a reduction in peak height velocity during puberty in both sexes, with early puberty occurring only in the girls.

Early or precocious puberty following the treatment of ALL with chemotherapy and cranial irradiation is well described (Leiper et al, 1988), and it is likely that abnormalities in the timing and tempo of puberty significantly contribute to the observed reduction in final height (Davies et al, 1994). A direct effect of chemotherapy on the spinal epiphyses is a possible explanation for the observed disproportion. However, a further factor contributing to the observed disproportion, more marked in the girls, may be an early puberty in combination with a reduced pubertal growth spurt (Didcock et al, 1995). If GH deficiency only becomes manifest during puberty in children who have received low-dose cranial irradiation (18–24 Gy), and spinal growth is an important and late part of the growth spurt, it is possible that disproportion may result. Skeletal disproportion, particularly in boys with precocious puberty, has been described (Martinez et al, 1984), but this is likely to be related to their underlying pathology, causing loss of consonance during pubertal growth. Interestingly, precocious puberty in the children treated for leukaemia occurs almost exclusively in the girls, whereas the observed skeletal disproportion is present in both sexes (Davies et al, 1995).

It is therefore likely that there is, in addition to GH insufficiency and disturbances in the timing of puberty, a direct effect of chemotherapy on the cartilaginous growth plate in children treated for ALL that contributes to the observed disproportion and the reduction in final height described by most authors.

Brain tumours

It is well recognized that the treatment of children with brain tumours with cranial irradiation doses in excess of 30 Gy results in GH deficiency and growth impairment. However, other factors are important in the aetiology of the growth failure, including spinal irradiation, poor nutrition, multiple pituitary hormone deficiency, early puberty and tumour recurrence. There is now increasing evidence that adjuvant chemotherapy is an important factor. A recent study of final height SDS in children treated for a brain tumour (Figure 2) showed a significant loss in final height SDS independent of age at irradiation in those children who received chemotherapy in addition to cranial irradiation (Ogilvy-Stuart and Shalet, 1995). Interestingly, the children treated with both cranial irradiation and chemotherapy did as badly in terms of overall stature as those who received craniospinal irradiation alone. The degree of disproportion following craniospinal irradiation is significantly greater than in the cranial irradiation group with chemotherapy, which suggests that the growth retardation observed involves the whole skeleton and is not confined to the spine. This is good evidence that factors other than a direct effect on spinal epiphyses are important in the observed disproportion in children treated for ALL. It may be that the observed effect of chemotherapy in these children is due to restrictive lung disease due to BCNU or CCNU restricting growth (O'Driscoll et al, 1990).

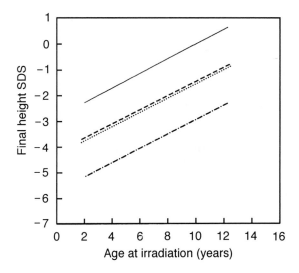

Figure 2. Parallel linear regression of final height SDS on age at irradiation according to the four treatment groups. Cranial irradiation alone (——), cranial irradiation plus chemotherapy (--------), craniospinal irradiation alone (·········), and craniospinal irradiation plus chemotherapy (-··-··-··-·). Reproduced from Ogilvy-Stuart and Shalet (1995, *Acta Pediatrica* **411**: 52–56) with permission.

Other tumours

Children with solid tumours not treated with cranial irradiation, and therefore not GH-insufficient, have also demonstrated catch-up growth following completion of chemotherapy (Glasser et al, 1991) but at final height were shown to be shorter than the normal population. The effect of actinomycin D has been shown to enhance the growth-retarding effect of irradiation in mice (Littman and D'Angio, 1979) and potentiates the loss in spinal height observed after abdominal irradiation in children treated for a Wilms' tumour (Wallace and Shalet, 1992).

In vitro studies

There is in vitro evidence for a direct effect of chemotherapy on the action of IGF-I at the cartilage growth plate and on the production of IGF-I by the liver (Morris, 1981). The effects of seven chemotherapeutic agents used in the treatment of leukaemia were studied in the isolated perfused rat liver and using a porcine costal cartilage bioassay. The uptake of [^{35}S]sulphate and [^{3}H]thymidine in the cartilage bioassay were both inhibited by prednisolone sodium sulphate and doxorubicin; 6-mercaptopurine, methotrexate and cyclophosphamide had no inhibitory effects, vincristine inhibited only [^{35}S]sulphate uptake and cytosine arabinoside inhibited only [^{3}H]thymidine uptake. In contrast, in the liver perfusion system, 6-mercaptopurine and vincristine rapidly inhibited IGF-I production, while cyclophosphamide and cytosine arabinoside caused a late and less pronounced decrease. These studies provide the only in vitro experimental evidence that chemotherapy has a profound effect on the IGF-I/chondrocyte axis.

Short-term growth

Knemometry

Knemometry is now recognized as the technique of choice for studying short-term growth (Valk et al, 1983; Wales and Milner, 1987) as it allows precise, reproducible, non-invasive measurements of lower leg length in growing children, such that daily (or even within-day) and weekly fluctuations in leg length can be recorded. It is not yet clear, however, whether short-term changes are due to changes in soft tissue composition or skeletal remodelling at the level of the growth plate. There have to date been two studies of short-term growth during treatment for ALL. Davies (1996) studied five patients during treatment for ALL over a median duration of 69 weeks and found that the normal episodic pattern of growth was preserved. In contrast, using a random zero method, which has been shown to reduce observer bias (Ahmed et al, 1995), we have found in two patients that lower leg length velocity mirrored changes in pro-collagen type I C-terminal pro-peptide (P1CP) and bone alkaline phosphatase (BALP) (see below). There was progressive slowing during induction and first intensification followed by catch-up, with further suppression and subsequent catch-up at second intensification. In both studies, there is a temporal relationship between episodes of neutropenic fever and reduced lower leg length velocity (Crofton et al, 1996a,b).

Biochemical markers

Carefully chosen biochemical markers of growth may overcome some of the disadvantages of knemometry. Knemometry ignores spinal growth and may be influenced by the hydration state of the soft tissues overlying the bone. In addition, knemometry is not possible in young children below about 4 years of age. Biochemical markers are free from observer bias, and their precision is independent of the frequency of sampling. BALP is found in the hypertrophic chondrocytes of the epiphyseal growth plate, in the matrix vesicles associated with bone mineralization and in mature osteoblasts. There is a close quantitative relationship between serial measurements of BALP and height velocity in short normal children undergoing GH treatment (Crofton et al 1995, 1996c).

P1CP is released into the circulation by proliferating osteoblasts during collagen biosynthesis. The cross-linked telopeptide of type I collagen (ICTP) is released into the circulation by collagen breakdown during bone modelling. Pro-collagen type III N-terminal pro-peptide (P3NP) is released during soft tissue growth but is not present in bone (see also Chapter 9 in this issue).

In a prospective longitudinal study of 12 children with ALL (Crofton et al 1996a,b), marked and significant changes in collagen pro-peptides and

BALP were seen during the first 6 months of chemotherapy (Figure 3). At diagnosis, P1CP and BALP were generally below or close to the lower limit of the reference range, suggesting impairment of bone growth by the disease process itself. During induction and first intensification, the collagen markers were progressively suppressed, whereas BALP showed initial recovery before subsequent suppression.

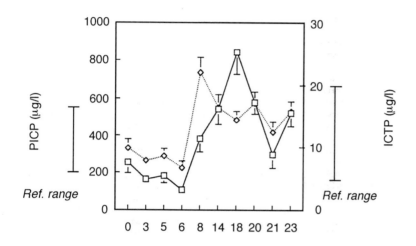

Treatment week

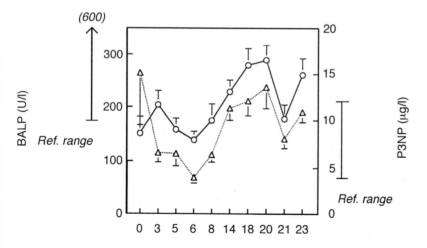

Treatment week

Figure 3. Biochemical markers of bone and growth in 12 patients (mean and SE). For abbreviations and explanation, see text. (—□—) PICP mean; (···◇···) ICTP mean; (—○—) BALP mean; (···△···) P3NP mean.

We postulate that these changes are due largely to the prednisolone component of chemotherapy, which was given continuously (40 mg/m^2, orally) throughout induction and first intensification. Glucocorticoids are known to have an inhibitory effect on collagen synthesis and degradation and on the cartilage zones of the growth plate (Cutroneo et al, 1981; Hill, 1981; Canalis, 1983) (see Chapter 7 in this issue). After first intensification (when prednisolone was withdrawn), a dramatic catch-up was observed in all bone markers, with the collagen markers reaching supranormal concentrations (paired t-tests $P<0.001$). During second intensification, all markers were again suppressed ($P<0.05$), followed by a second catch-up ($P<0.05$) (Crofton et al 1996a,b).

It remains to be determined whether the degree of marker suppression or the adequacy of marker catch-up have any predictive value for assessing outcome in terms of height deficit or subsequent growth. Continuing studies of markers of GH secretion (urinary GH, IGF-I and IGFBP-3) should help further to identify whether the pattern of growth is mediated through GH secretion or is a direct effect on target tissues.

THYROID

There is little evidence that chemotherapy *per se* causes thyroid dysfunction; the most important agent responsible for thyroid dysfunction is radiation to the neck region. However, there is evidence that the effect of radiotherapy on the thyroid may be potentiated by chemotherapy (Livesey and Brook, 1989). In this study of 119 survivors who had been treated for a brain tumour, thyroid dysfunction was found in 11 out of 47 children who had received spinal irradiation but no chemotherapy, and in 20 out of 29 patients who had received spinal irradiation and chemotherapy. These findings were confirmed by a study from Manchester (Ogilvy-Stuart et al, 1991), which also studied thyroid dysfunction after treatment of brain tumours. Interestingly, there was a significant increase in compensated thyroid dysfunction in children receiving adjuvant cytotoxic chemotherapy. Not surprisingly, there was a significantly higher incidence of thyroid dysfunction after craniospinal irradiation than after cranial irradiation. Of particular interest is the finding that the speed of onset of thyroid dysfunction is accelerated when adjuvant chemotherapy is administered.

The most common abnormality was compensated thyroid dysfunction, with a raised thyroid-stimulating hormone (TSH) concentration and a normal free T4. It seems sensible to treat with T4 those children who have hyperthyrotropinaemia, even in the presence of a normal T4 level, to return the serum TSH level to normal and thus reduce the theoretical risk of thyroid cancer (Field et al, 1978).

GONADAL DYSFUNCTION

The impact of combination cytotoxic chemotherapy on gonadal function is dependent on the nature and dosage of the drugs received by the child.

Drugs that have been shown to cause gonadal damage include the alkylating agents, such as cyclophosphamide, chlorambucil and the nitrosoureas, in addition to procarbazine, vinblastine, cytosine arabinoside and possibly cis-platinum (Wallace et al, 1989).

Just as is seen in girls with Turner syndrome, it is frequently impossible to detect biochemically cytotoxic-induced gonadal damage during prepubertal life, abnormally elevated gonadotrophin levels occurring only when the child has reached an age at which the onset of puberty would have been expected.

Testis

The adult male testis has two important functions: spermatogenesis and steroidogenesis. The Sertoli cells are intimately involved in supporting the maturation of germ cells into spermatozoa within the seminiferous tubules. In addition, Sertoli cells produce many proteins, including an androgen-binding protein that binds testosterone and is important for normal spermatogenesis. The androgen testosterone is necessary for the development of secondary sex characteristics and is synthesized within the Leydig cells situated in the interstitium of the testis. The production of testosterone by the Leydig cells is under the control of the hypothalamic–pituitary axis. The assessment of testicular function requires pubertal staging, including measuring testicular volumes, basal levels of follicle-stimulating hormone (FSH), luteinizing hormone (LH) and testosterone, and semen analysis if appropriate.

Acute lymphoblastic leukaemia (ALL)

Lendon et al (1978) studied testicular histology after testicular biopsy in 44 boys treated with combination chemotherapy for ALL. The tubular fertility index (TFI) was calculated as the percentage of tubules containing identifiable spermatogonia. The mean TFI was 50% of that in age-matched controls, and 18 of the biopsies had a severely depressed TFI of 40% or less. Three variables had a highly significant effect on the TFI. Previous chemotherapy with cyclophosphamide or cytosine arabinoside depressed the TFI, whereas with increasing time after completion of chemotherapy, the TFI improved.

In a prospective study of 14 boys with ALL (Blatt et al, 1981) who were treated with a combination of vincristine, prednisolone, methotrexate and 6-mercaptopurine, normal testicular function was documented through puberty as determined by normal testicular maturation and appropriate gonadotrophin and serum testosterone levels. Semen analysis was normal in the six boys studied. Not surprisingly, testicular function was normal as the chemotherapy did not include drugs known to cause testicular damage.

In an Australian study of testicular function in 25 boys treated with a modified lymphosarcoma 2 lymphoma 2 (LSA_2L_2) protocol (Quigley et al, 1989) that consisted of 10 cytotoxic agents including cyclophosphamide and cytosine arabinoside, given for 3 or 4 years, severe testicular damage was reported. In 24 testicular biopsies assessed at the time of completion of chemotherapy, there was an absence of germ cells in 13, and in the remaining 11 the germ cells were markedly depleted. Elevation of the basal FSH and an exaggerated FSH response to an acute bolus of gonadotrophin-releasing hormone (GnRH) were reported in the majority of boys who were pubertal at assessment. Furthermore, all 13 pubertal boys had pathologically small testes for their pubertal stage.

To assess the reversibility of documented germ cell damage after chemotherapy for ALL in childhood, testicular function was studied in 37 long-term survivors (Wallace et al, 1991). This study was conducted at two separate time points; initially, a wedge testicular biopsy was performed at or near completion of chemotherapy to assess the incidence of occult testicular relapse. The TFI was calculated then and subsequently at a median time of 10.7 years after stopping chemotherapy; the patients were re-assessed by clinical examination, measurement of gonadotrophins and testosterone levels and, in 19, by semen analysis. The median TFI for all 37 biopsies was 74%, and at reassessment six men had evidence of severe damage to the germinal epithelium. Five men had azoospermia and one had a reduced mean testicular volume and a raised basal FSH concentration consistent with severe germ cell damage. Of 11 males who had a TFI less than 50% at testicular biopsy, five recovered normal germ cell function at a median of 10.1 years after chemotherapy.

The current management of ALL in children in the UK includes cytosine arabinoside for all patients and cyclophosphamide for those who are randomized to receive a third intensification block of treatment. The long-term outlook for fertility for this group of patients is not yet known. However, the available evidence suggests that current treatment regimens used in the UK are unlikely to be sterilizing and the vast majority of survivors will not require androgen treatment to achieve normal virilization and sexual function. Those patients who have required testicular irradiation as part of their treatment are, however, highly likely to be sterile and require androgen replacement therapy for life.

Hodgkin's disease

The first report of chemotherapy-induced testicular damage in patients treated for Hodgkin's disease in childhood with MOPP (nitrogen mustard, vincristine, procarbazine and prednisolone) (Sherins et al, 1978) demonstrated that the majority of pubertal boys had a raised basal FSH level, and all of those who had testicular biopsies had germinal aplasia. Chemotherapy with MOPP in children was also shown to cause damage to the germinal epithelium, resulting in azoospermia between 2.4 and 8 years after completion of chemotherapy (Whitehead et al, 1982a).

In adult males treated for Hodgkin's disease with six or more courses of MVPP (mustine, vinblastine, procarbazine and prednisolone), azoospermia is the rule and recovery of spermatogenesis with increasing time after completion of chemotherapy rare (Whitehead et al, 1982b). In a recent study (Mackie et al, 1996) of 101 post-pubertal subjects, all of whom had received ChLVPP (chlorambucil, vinblastine, procarbazine and pred-nisolone) in childhood with no radiotherapy below the diaphragm, 89% had evidence of severe damage to the germinal epithelium with raised basal FSH levels. Interestingly, subtle Leydig cell dysfunction was identified in 24%, with raised LH levels and a serum testosterone within the normal range. All patients progressed spontaneously through puberty but require long-term follow-up as Leydig cell function may become compromised, with implications for bone mineralization in young adulthood and normal sexual function.

These studies have clearly indicated that the pre-pubertal testis is not protected from chemotherapy potentially toxic to the gonads and that pre- and peri-pubertal FSH estimations are unreliable in predicting testicular damage (Wallace, 1996).

Ovary

The interpretation of tests of ovarian function in women treated for cancer in childhood is difficult. A regular menstrual cycle and normal adult secondary sexual characteristics are likely to be associated with normal fertility. Menstrual irregularity and minor abnormalities of basal and stimulated gonadotrophins do not preclude the potential for fertility. The assessment of ovarian function should include a menstrual history and the assessment of secondary sexual characteristics. The measurement of basal gonadotrophins and serum oestradiol is helpful, and the measurement of luteal phase progesterone may confirm that the cycles are ovulatory. Further assessment may include pelvic ultrasound examination of ovarian and uterine size and endometrial thickness (Critchley et al, 1992).

Acute lymphoblastic leukaemia (ALL)

The majority of early reports of ovarian function in children treated with combination chemotherapy for ALL suggest that ovarian damage is un-common (Siris et al, 1976; Pasqualini et al, 1987; Green et al, 1989). However, Quigley et al (1989) found significantly higher basal and peak FSH levels following GnRH administration in pre-pubertal and pubertal girls treated with a modified LSA_2L_2 protocol than in controls; despite this, all girls reached puberty at a normal time and had normal oestradiol levels. In a recent UK study of 40 girls treated in childhood for ALL, all achieved adult pubertal development and 37 had regular menses. There were 14 live births in nine long-term survivors, with no serious congenital abnormalities and no reported cases of malignant disease (Wallace et al, 1993). Modern treatment for ALL in the UK seems unlikely to be sterilizing, although these women may be at increased risk of a premature menopause.

Hodgkin's disease

There are few reports of ovarian function following the treatment of Hodgkin's disease in childhood. Although an early report (Bramswig et al,

1989) suggested that ovarian function was normal in all women studied, a recent British study of women treated with ChLVPP and no below-diaphragm radiotherapy demonstrated raised gonadotrophin levels with variable oestradiol levels in 53% (Mackie et al, 1996). Further follow-up of these women is clearly required to determine whether there is recovery of ovarian function or whether progression to a premature menopause is inevitable. In this study, 7 women have achieved 11 normal pregnancies, and 2 of these women had raised gonadotrophins before conception. Reassuringly, there is no evidence in the literature of an increased risk of miscarriage following chemotherapy or an increased number of abnormalities in the offspring.

OBESITY

There is a clinical impression that survivors of ALL and brain tumours are obese following treatment. A recent study (Didi et al, 1995) identified two main factors associated with an increased body mass index following treatment for ALL. Female gender and younger age at diagnosis were both associated, but neither could be used to predict obesity at final height. Girls treated for ALL became obese during treatment, after which there was no further increase, and there was no correlation with GH insufficiency, disproportionate growth or abnormalities in the timing of puberty. There is evidence that chemotherapy has an effect on substrate utilization, causing inhibition of fat oxidation in the fasting state, which has been attributed to the use of steroids (Stallings et al, 1989). Patients treated for ALL receive 5-day, monthly pulsed doses of steroids for at least 2 years; it is therefore likely that steroids play an important part in the development of obesity. However this would not explain the observed gender differences, which may be reflected in other factors such as diminished exercise capacity or opportunity.

SUMMARY

With the move away from radiotherapy in the treatment of children with ALL and young children with brain tumours, the potential short- and long-term effects of chemotherapy are receiving increasing attention. Gonadal dysfunction following chemotherapy is well recognized, but the effects of chemotherapy on growth may be more subtle and no less important. In vivo and in vitro studies have provided strong evidence for a direct effect of chemotherapy on the growth plate. Glucocorticoids, in particular, may be important in both the growth failure and obesity that are now well described following treatment for ALL. Thyroid dysfunction is an inevitable consequence of direct radiotherapy, but chemotherapy may potentiate these effects. Further studies of short-term growth, as measured by knemometry and using biochemical markers of bone and collagen turnover, will provide further insight into the mechanisms of growth failure, which will be important in the design of the next generation of anti-cancer treatments.

REFERENCES

Ahmed SF, Wallace WHB & Kelnar CJH (1995) Knemometry in childhood: a study to compare the precision of two different techniques. *Annals of Human Biology* **22:** 247–252.

Blatt J, Poplack DG & Sherins RJ (1981) Testicular function after chemotherapy for acute lymphoblastic leukaemia. *New England Journal of Medicine* **304:** 1121–1124.

Bramswig JH, Heiermann E, Heimes U et al (1989) Ovarian function in 63 girls treated for Hodgkin's disease according to the West-German DAL-HD-78 and DAL-HD-82 therapy study. *Medical and Paediatric Oncology* **17:** 344.

Canalis E (1983) Effect of glucocorticoids on type 1 collagen synthesis, alkaline phosphatase activity and deoxyribonucleic acid content in cultured rat calvariae. *Endocrinology* **112:** 931–939.

Clayton PE, Shalet SM, Morris-Jones PH & Price DA (1988) Growth in children treated for acute lymphoblastic leukaemia. *Lancet* **i:** 460–462.

Critchley HOD, Wallace WHB, Mamtora H et al (1992) Ovarian failure after whole abdominal radiotherapy; the potential for pregnancy. *British Journal of Obstetrics and Gynaecology* **99:** 3392–3394.

Crofton PM, Stirling HF & Kelnar CJH (1995) Bone alkaline phosphatase and height velocity in short normal children undergoing growth-promoting treatments: a longitudinal study. *Clinical Chemistry* **41:** 672–678.

Crofton PM, Stirling HF, Schonau E & Kelnar CJH (1996c) Bone alkaline phosphatase and collagen markers as early predictors of height velocity response to growth-promoting treatments in short normal children. *Clinical Endocrinology* (in press).

Crofton PM, Stirling HF, Schonau E et al (1996a) Collagen markers and bone alkaline phosphatase as predictors of bone turnover and growth. Excerpta Medica International Congress Series. Amsterdam: Excerpta Medica (in press).

Crofton PM, Stirling HF, Schonau E et al (1996b) Biochemical markers of bone turnover. *Hormone Research* (in press).

Crowne EC, Moore C, Wallace WHB et al (1992) A novel variant of growth hormone insufficiency following low dose cranial irradiation. *Clinical Endocrinology* **36:** 59–68.

Cutroneo KR, Rokowski R & Counts DF (1981) Glucocorticoids and collagen synthesis: comparison of in vivo and cell culture studies. *Collagen Rel Research* **1:** 557–568.

Davies HA (1996) Treatment for lymphoblastic leukaemia in childhood: effects on growth and puberty. MD Thesis, University of Bristol.

Davies HA, Didcock E, Didi M et al (1994) Disproportionate short stature after cranial irradiation and combination chemotherapy for leukaemia. *Archives of Disease in Childhood* **70:** 472–475.

Davies HA, Didcock E, Didi M et al (1995) Growth puberty and obesity after treatment for leukaemia. *Acta Pediatrica* **411 supplement:** 45–50.

Didcock E, Davies HA, Didi M (1995) Pubertal growth in young adult survivors of childhood leukaemia. *Journal of Clinical Oncology* **13:** 2503–2507.

Didi M, Didcock E, Davies HA et al (1995) High incidence of obesity in young adults after treatment of acute lymphoblastic leukaemia in childhood. *Journal of Pediatrics* **127:** 63–67.

Field JB, Bloom G, Chou MCY et al (1978) Effect of thyroid stimulating hormone on human thyroid carcinoma and adjacent normal tissue. *Journal of Clinical Endocrinology and Metabolism* **47:** 1052–1058.

Glasser DB, Duane K, Lane JM et al (1991) The effect of chemotherapy on growth in the skeletally immature individual. *Clinical Orthopedics* **262:** 101–107.

Green DM, Hall B & Zevon A (1989) Pregnancy outcome after treatment for acute lymphoblastic leukaemia during childhood or adolescence. *Cancer* **64:** 2335–2339.

Hill DJ (1981) Effects of cortisol on cell proliferation and proteoglycan synthesis and degradation in cartilage zones of the calf costochondral growth plate in vitro with and without rat plasma somatomedin activity. *Journal of Endocrinology* **88:** 425–435.

Hokken-Keolega ACS, Van Doorn JWD, Hahlen K et al (1993) Long-term effects of treatment for acute lymphoblastic leukaemia with and without cranial irradiation on growth and puberty: a comparative study. *Pediatric Research* **33:** 577–582.

Holm K, Nysom K, Hertz H & Muller J (1994) Normal final height after treatment for acute lymphoblastic leukaemia without irradiation. *Acta Pediatrica Scandinavica* **83:** 1287–1290.

Katz JA, Chambers B, Everhart C et al (1991) Linear growth in children with acute lymphoblastic leukaemia treated without cranial irradiation. *Journal of Pediatrics* **118:** 575–578.

Kirk JA, Raghupathy P, Stevens MM et al (1987) Growth failure and growth-hormone deficiency after treatment for acute lymphoblastic leukaemia. *Lancet* **i:** 190–193.

Leiper AD, Stanhope R, Preece MA et al (1988) Precocious or early puberty and growth failure in girls treated for acute lymphoblastic leukaemia. *Hormone Research* **30:** 72–76.

Lendon M, Hann IM, Palmer MK et al (1978) Testicular histology after combination chemotherapy in childhood for acute lymphoblastic leukaemia. *Lancet* **ii:** 439–441.

Littman PS & D'Angio GJ (1979) Growth considerations in the radiation therapy of children with cancer. *Annual Review of Medicine* **30:** 405–415.

Livesey EA & Brook CGD (1989) Thyroid dysfunction after radiotherapy and chemotherapy of brain tumours. *Archives of Disease in Childhood* **64:** 593–595.

Mackie EJ, Radford M & Shalet SM (1996) Gonadal function following chemotherapy for childhood Hodgkin's disease. *Medical and Paediatric Oncology* (in press).

Martinez L, Preece MA & Grant DB (1984) Body proportions in precocious puberty. *Acta Pediatrica* **73:** 185–188.

Moell C, Garwicz S, Westgren U et al (1988) Blunted pubertal growth after leukaemia: a new pattern of growth hormone insufficiency. *Hormone Research* **30:** 68–71.

Moell C, Marky I, Hovi L et al (1994) Cerebral irradiation causes blunted pubertal growth in girls treated for acute leukaemia. *Medical and Pediatric Oncology* **22:** 375–379.

Mohnike K, Timme J, Kluba U et al (1995) Growth and puberty in children with acute lymphoblastic leukaemia treated with two different chemotherapeutic protocols. *Acta Pediatrica* **(supplement):** 100.

Morris MJ (1981) In vitro effects of anti-leukaemic drugs on cartilage metabolism and their effects on somatomedin production by the liver. PhD thesis, Manchester University.

O'Driscoll BR, Hasleton PS, Taylor PM et al (1990) Active lung fibrosis up to 17 years after chemotherapy with carmustine (BCNU) in childhood. *New England Journal of Medicine* **323:** 378–382.

Ogilvy-Stuart AL & Shalet SM (1995) Effect of chemotherapy on growth. *Acta Pediatrica* **411: (Supplement):** 52–56.

Ogilvy-Stuart AL, Shalet SM & Gattamaneni HR (1991) Thyroid function after treatment of brain tumours in children. *Journal of Pediatrics* **119:** 733–737.

Pasqualini T, Escobar ME, Domene H et al (1987) Evaluation of gonadal function following long-term treatment for acute lymphoblastic leukaemia in girls. *American Journal of Pediatric Hematology and Oncology* **9:** 115–122.

Quigley C, Cowell C, Jimenez M et al (1989) Normal or early development of puberty despite gonadal damage in children treated for acute lymphoblastic leukaemia. *New England Journal of Medicine* **321:** 143–151.

Shalet SM, Price DA, Beardwell CG et al (1979) Normal growth despite abnormalities of growth hormone secretion in children treated for acute leukaemia. *Journal of Pediatrics* **94:** 719–722.

Sherins RJ, Olweny CLM & Ziegler JL (1978) Gynaecomastia and gonadal dysfunction in adolescent boys treated with combination chemotherapy for Hodgkin's disease. *New England Journal of Medicine* **299:** 12–16.

Siris ES, Leventhal BG & Vaitukaitis JL (1976) Effects of childhood leukaemia and chemotherapy on puberty and reproductive function in girls. *New England Journal of Medicine* **294:** 1143–1146.

Sklar C, Mertens A, Walter A et al (1993) Final height after treatment of acute lymphoblastic leukaemia: a comparison of no cranial irradiation, 1800 cGy and 2400 cGy cranial irradiation. *Journal of Pediatrics* **123:** 59–64.

Stalling VA, Vaisman N, Chan HSL et al (1989) Energy metabolism in children with newly diagnosed acute lymphoblastic leukaemia. *Pediatric Research* **26:** 154–157.

Valk IM, Langhout-Chabloz AME, Smals AGH et al (1983) Accurate measurement of the lower leg length and ulnar length and its application in short term growth measurement. *Growth* **47:** 53–66.

Wales JKH & Milner RDG (1987) Knemometry in the assessment of linear growth. *Archives of Disease in Childhood* **62:** 166–171.

Wallace WHB (1996) Growth and endocrine function following treatment of childhood malignant disease. In Plowman PN & Pinkerton CR (eds) *Paediatric Oncology: Clinical Practice and Controversies.* London: Chapman & Hall (in press).

Wallace WHB & Shalet SM (1992) Chemotherapy with actinomycin D influences the growth of the spine following abdominal irradiation. *Medical and Pediatric Encology* **20:** 177 (letter).

Wallace WHB, Shalet SM, Lendon M & Morris-Jones PH (1991) Male fertility in long-term survivors of acute lymphoblastic leukaemia in childhood. *International Journal of Andrology* **14:** 312–319.

Wallace WHB, Shalet SM, Tetlow LJ & Morris-Jones PH (1993) Ovarian function following the treatment of childhood acute lymphoblastic leukaemia. *Medical and Pediatric Oncology* **21:** 333–339.

Wallace WHB, Shalet SM, Crowne EC et al (1989) Gonadal dysfunction due to cis-platinum. *Medical and Pediatric Oncology* **17:** 409–413.

Whitehead E, Shalet SM, Morris-Jones PH et al (1982a) Gonadal function after combination chemotherapy for Hodgkin's disease in childhood. *Archives of Disease in Childhood* **57:** 287–291.

Whitehead E, Shalet SM, Blackledge G et al (1982b) The effects of Hodgkin's disease and combination chemotherapy on gonadal function in the adult male. *Cancer* **49:** 418–422.

8

Bone mineralization at puberty: clinical relevance for health and disease

ASAD RAHIM
SARAH J. HOLMES
STEPHEN M. SHALET

At puberty, marked changes in the skeleton occur, which include growth and ossification. These skeletal changes may have far-reaching consequences, particularly with regard to the development of osteoporosis in adulthood, as the rate of bone mineralization and bone mass accretion are maximal during puberty. In young women, bone mineral accretion begins with the onset of puberty and continues until the age of 16 years, or 2 years after menarche, and in men it usually continues until the age of 20 years (Glastre et al, 1990; Bonjour et al, 1991; Katzman et al, 1991). This conclusion is supported by a longitudinal study (Theintz et al, 1992) in which bone mass accumulation was demonstrated to be maximal between the ages of 13 and 17 years in young men, and 11 and 14 years in young girls. During the age period 17–20 years, although there was an increase in bone mass, this was not significant. Associated with maximal bone mass accumulation is the fact that more than half of the bone calcium is normally laid down during this period.

BONE STRUCTURE

Normal bone has two main components: cortical (compact) bone and cancellous (trabecular) bone. At various sites, a combination of these types of bone exists, and this is known as integral bone.

Cortical bone comprises 80% of the total skeleton. Bone turnover in this region is much slower, making it more stable than trabecular bone.

Trabecular bone is composed of connecting plates of bone that contain multiple holes, giving it a porous appearance. It is within this trabecular bone that many of the active metabolic processes concerned with bone formation occur, and with the increased surface area, bone turnover is about eight times greater than that of cortical bone. Certain regions of the skeleton are richer in trabecular bone. These include the vertebrae, the femoral necks and the distal radii. As a result of being more metabolically

Baillière's Clinical Paediatrics—
Vol. 4, No. 2, May 1996
ISBN 0–7020–2180–6
0963–6714/96/020349 + 16 $12.00/00

active, it is trabecular bone that is more readily affected by pathological conditions. It is therefore not surprising that pathological conditions often manifest as fractures of the vertebrae, hip and wrist.

Within bone there are four types of cells present: osteoblasts, osteoclasts, resting surface cells and osteocytes.

Osteoblasts are polyhedral cells that cover the surface of trabecular bone in their resting state. It is these cells that are mainly responsible for new bone formation. They are also responsible for active calcification and mineralization of newly formed bone. Osteoblasts eventually become either incorporated into mineralized bone matrix, lose many of their organelles and become osteocytes, or become flatter and cover resting bone surfaces as resting surface cells.

Osteocytes are small cells that lie in lacunae filled by interstitial fluid surrounded by mineralized bone matrix. The function of the fluid is to allow transfer of metabolites to and from the mineralized matrix. It is believed that through this route osteocytes may play a role in matrix metabolism.

Osteoclasts are thought to originate from haemopoietic stem cells and are responsible for bone resorption. Resorption of bone is the process of removal of mineral and organic matrix from bone. It is necessary for bone remodelling (the process of controlled replacement of old matrix by new) and the maintenance of serum calcium levels.

The development and modelling of bone is a process that is controlled by hormones and growth factors. Growth factors are made by several tissues and are present in both the systemic circulation and the bone matrix. Other growth factors are made by skeletal cells; these include insulin-like growth factors-I and -II (IGF-I and II), transforming growth factor-β (TGF-β) and certain bone morphogenic proteins (BMPs). Hormones which principally affect skeletal development during puberty are sex steroids and growth hormone (GH).

The increase in GH and IGF-I levels during puberty is associated with markedly increased osteoblastic activity and number, resulting in bone growth. This growth is mediated by both GH directly and also IGF-I, which is produced both systemically and locally. The increased number and activity of osteoblasts that occurs as a consequence of increased levels of GH results in increased bone mineral deposition. This in turn increases overall bone mineral density.

During puberty, the accumulation of bone mass increases by between four-fold and six-fold over a 3-year period in girls and a 4-year period in boys (Bonjour et al, 1994). This increase is measurable at both the lumbar spine and femoral neck, areas that are richer in the more metabolically active trabecular bone. The equilibrium of activity reached by osteoblasts and osteoclasts is responsible for the maintenance of skeletal structure and should be achieved once peak bone mass is attained. This is usually several years after puberty is complete.

From an organic perspective, bone is composed of an osteoid and minerals (mainly calcium and phosphate). Although there are 15 different types of collagen, the principle one in bone is type I collagen. Collagen, along with several other matrix materials, forms the base upon which calcium and phosphate are deposited. The mechanisms of bone mineralization are not fully understood.

FACTORS INFLUENCING BONE MINERALIZATION AND THE ATTAINMENT OF PEAK BONE MASS

Genetic factors

Genetic factors have a very large influence on the attainment of peak bone mass. Women whose mothers develop post-menopausal osteoporosis are more likely to develop clinically significant bone disease in adulthood. The bone mass and bone mineral density of children closely resembles that of their parents, and that of identical twins correlates more closely than does that of non-identical twins.

Racial origin and ethnicity also influence bone mass (Politzer and Anderson, 1989; Patel et al, 1993). Black children have been shown to have a greater mean bone mineral density than their white counterparts.

Body mass

Increased body mass is associated with increased bone mass. This is probably due to increased mechanical loading on the skeleton, but increased body mass also suggests better nutrition. Using the twin model, however, Young et al (1995) showed that lean body mass rather than fat mass was the more important determinant of bone mass in girls and young women.

Calcium intake

In the process of growth, total body calcium increases from around 30 g at birth to 1300 g at maturity. This is nearly all contained within the skeleton, so a mean calcium requirement of 175 mg per day is needed for development of the skeleton over 20 years of growth.

Recently, the effect of calcium supplementation on bone mass in adolescence has been studied. Elegant experiments using twin pairs to exclude genetic influences have shown that, at least in pre-pubertal children, the administration of calcium supplements was beneficial to the skeleton (Johnston et al, 1992). After puberty, the differences were much less clear cut. A subsequent study confined to adolescent girls showed a beneficial effect of calcium supplementation whatever the pubertal status (Lloyd et al, 1993).

In a meta-analysis of calcium balance studies performed in subjects up to 30 years of age, Matkovic and Heaney (1992) showed a threshold effect above which a further increase in calcium intake led to no improvement in calcium retention. Although these thresholds vary with age, they are all in excess of the US recommended dietary allowances for calcium, suggesting that we should be considering a higher intake of calcium at times of skeletal growth.

Hormonal influences

GH has numerous effects on skeletal development. These include stimulation of the number and activity of osteoblasts, longitudinal bone growth
and the deposition of bone minerals.

GH release during childhood occurs in discrete pulses, predominantly
after the onset of sleep. The pattern and rate of GH release in both boys and
girls in the pre-pubertal period is very similar. Pre-pubertal boys and girls
have a mean GH secretion rate of about 0.6 U (20 mU/kg) during a 24-hour
period. However, changes in GH secretion occurring at puberty are sex
specific. In girls, increased GH secretion occurs at an earlier age than in
boys. However, GH secretory rate is maximal in boys and girls
(Albertsson-Wikland et al, 1994) during the same stage of puberty (Tanner
stage 4).

GH has a direct effect on bone growth, causing an increase in the length
of longitudinal bone. This arises from growth at the epiphyseal growth
plates. GH also acts indirectly via IGF-I. Systemic IGF-I is produced
predominantly by the liver and is GH-dependent. Systemic IGF-I acts on
cartilage, resulting in growth. Levels of systemic IGF-I increase during
puberty and usually reach their peak 1 year after peak growth velocity is
achieved. IGF-I levels then remain elevated for 4 further years, despite the
fact that the growth rate is decreasing.

Prior to puberty, sex steroids play a small role in growth and skeletal
development. However, with the increase in sex steroid levels during
puberty, their role becomes far more significant, especially during the
pubertal growth spurt. It is at this time that the rate of maximum accumulation of bone mass occurs. The timing of maximum accumulation of bone
mass appears to differ in males and females (Glastre et al, 1990). In males,
the greatest accumulation of bone mass in the lumbar spine and femoral
necks occurs between the ages of 13 and 17. In females, the maximum
increase in bone mass at these sites occurs earlier, between the ages of 11
and 14, and falls dramatically by 2 years after menarche (Theintz et al,
1992). The delay in the accumulation of lumbar spine bone mass in boys
has been attributed to the later age of onset of puberty in boys, suggesting
that the timing of the increase in circulating sex steroid levels is important
in the timing of peak acquisition of bone mass.

However, even at the end of puberty, bone mineral density is roughly
14% lower than the peak mass in young adults (Glastre et al, 1990), indicating that other factors also play a role in peak bone mass attainment and that
accumulation of bone mass continues for several years after the end of
puberty.

Although GH and sex steroids appear to have independent effects on
bone mass, sex steroids can influence circulating levels of GH and IGF-I,
suggesting that an interaction between these hormones may be important in
the acquisition and maintenance of bone mass. In addition, there is
evidence to suggest that GH has some gonadotrophic effects (Mason et al,
1990; Stanhope et al, 1991; Inzucchi and Robbins, 1994). This is further
supported by evidence that children with GH deficiency (Bourguignon et

al, 1986) and with GH insensitivity (Rosenfeld et al, 1994) show delayed pubertal development. During puberty, circulating testosterone and oestradiol concentrations increase. These are associated with an increase in endogenous pulsatile GH secretion in both males and females (Martha and Riggs, 1991). Even in adult life, endogenous oestradiol levels are a major influence on circulating GH levels, and variations in circulating levels of GH have been accounted for by variations in circulating levels of oestradiol in women and in young, compared with old, subjects (Ho et al, 1987). In men, serum testosterone levels are also positively correlated with spontaneous GH secretion (Iranmanesh et al, 1991; Corpas et al, 1992). In peripubertal boys (Rosenfield and Furlanetto, 1985) and men with idiopathic hypogonadotrophic hypogonadism (Liu et al, 1987), administration of testosterone enhances GH secretion.

ASSESSMENT OF BONE MINERALIZATION

Methods of bone density measurement

Assessment of bone mineral density in children is difficult for two main innate reasons. First, each of the techniques used has inate limitations. Second, the measurements being performed are in rapidly growing individuals, which means that there is a large variation in the normal range.

Methods used include quantitative computer tomography (QCT), single photon absorptiometry (SPA) and dual-energy X-ray absorptiometry (DXA).

QCT includes two methods, using either single-energy or dual-energy QCT. Both methods measure trabecular bone, scanning a mid-plane through each of four vertebrae. Dual-energy QCT is used to exclude apparent changes in bone mineral density due to marrow fat. QCT studies have been performed in pre-pubertal as well as pubertal children and have shown an increase in bone density in the latter group (Gilsanz et al, 1988). The technique of QCT is not subject to the confounding effect of bone size as it measures a volume of bone that is not influenced by the size of the patient.

Using QCT, it has also been shown that there is no difference in vertebral bone density between boys and girls once pubertal staging has been taken into account (Gilsanz et al, 1988).

SPA measures forearm bone mineral content at two sites. The more proximal site measures cortical bone, and the ultradistal site measures cortical and trabecular bone. SPA involves an area measurement, i.e. the amount of bone mineral per unit length, which is therefore dependent on the size of forearm bones. Even if SPA length is standardized, the volume of bone will be greater in a big child than in a small child. This measurement is therefore limited by the fact that it is taking place in a growing child and also by the fact that children of the same age and pubertal stage may be different sizes. This may incorrectly suggest a reduced bone mineral density and bone mass in the smallest children. Studies utilizing SPA have shown an increase in bone mass with age and have also in adolescents revealed a larger amount of bone mass in boys compared with girls (Foresta et al, 1983a,b). This is probably related to increased stature in boys compared with girls, rather than being a true difference in bone mass.

DXA measures integral bone. Measurements are of bone in the whole body and selected anatomical sites, which include the lumbar spine (L_2–L_4) and right femoral neck. This technique is useful in children as it involves minimal radiation exposure, short scanning time, high accuracy and high precision (Glastre et al, 1990).

Markers of bone turnover

A number of markers for bone metabolism exist (Eriksen et al, 1995). Some reflect bone formation and may be osteoblast products or byproducts of collagen precursors. Certain products of bone and collagen degradation can also be measured and used as markers of bone resorption.

Alkaline phosphatase comes from several sources, including the liver, intestine and bone. In children, the main source of alkaline phosphatase is bone, and the majority of bone alkaline phosphatase is derived from osteoblasts. Osteocalcin, like alkaline phosphatase, is also produced by osteoblasts. Both osteocalcin and bone alkaline phosphatase reflect bone formation.

Carboxy-terminal pro-peptide of type I collagen (PICP) is cleaved from pro-collagen before it is incorporated into collagen fibrils. It has been shown to be a sensitive marker of bone metabolism, especially bone formation.

Hydroxyproline is an amino acid that is present in collagen and is released from bone matrix during collagen breakdown. This is not re-used and is excreted in the urine, where it can be measured. Urinary levels of hydroxyproline, however, also reflect the turnover of extraskeletal collagens, so are not specific for bone resorption. The urinary hydroxyproline measurement is also affected by dietary absorption of hydroxyproline. Despite these limitations, the measurement of urinary hydroxyproline represents a useful indicator of bone resorption if used in association with other markers of bone turnover.

Deoxypyridinoline is found almost exclusively in bone and dentin. It is a byproduct of bone resorption that is excreted in the urine. It is a specific and accurate marker of bone resorption.

Carboxy-terminal telopeptide type I collagen (ITCP) is found in bone and cartilage and is released during bone resorption. It remains stable in the serum and is not degraded, which allows it to be used as a sensitive marker of bone resorption.

Biochemical markers of bone turnover, such as osteocalcin, alkaline phosphatase and urinary deoxypyridinoline, have been shown to correlate with circulating GH and IGF-I levels during puberty. These markers indicate that bone turnover, and therefore bone mineral deposition, is highest in mid-puberty and decreases towards adult levels in late puberty (Blumsohn et al, 1994). Blumsohn et al (1994) also found that levels of PICP and ICTP, although raised, were not as high as other markers. This suggested that these markers were possibly less sensitive indicators of skeletal health during puberty.

Markers for bone resorption and bone formation increase in parallel during puberty. Although puberty is principally a time of bone formation rather than resorption, there is much bone remodelling during this period. Thus the processes of bone formation and resorption are occurring simultaneously, which accounts for the parallel increase of both sets of markers.

GH DEFICIENCY

Isolated GH deficiency usually presents with slow growth in children before they reach puberty, which is typically delayed in onset. Bone mass in these children with GH deficiency in childhood has been shown to be significantly reduced compared with normal control subjects (Shore et al, 1980; Zamboni et al, 1991; Saggese et al, 1993); however, the techniques used for these observations are limited in growing children. Another study (Degerblad et al, 1992) reported that adults with childhood-onset GH deficiency have reduced forearm cortical and integral bone mass compared with men and women of approximately the same age. However, this group did not comment on the statistical significance of this finding, and the number of subjects in this study was small. Others later reported a significant reduction in bone mass in adults with childhood-onset GH deficiency (Hyer et al, 1992; Kaufman et al, 1992; Amato et al, 1993; O'Halloran et al, 1993; De Boer et al, 1994). Kaufman et al (1992) reported a 20–30% reduction in bone mineral density in the forearm and one of between 9 and 19% in the lumbar spine. Follow-up in these cases suggested that the reduction in bone mineral density was due to a failure of bone mass accretion during the pubertal growth spurt rather than to premature bone loss during adulthood. Hyer et al (1992) used DXA to demonstrate that untreated GH deficiency during puberty resulted in reduced bone mineral density compared with age-matched, healthy controls. This group (Hyer et al, 1992) also showed that GH-deficient patients who did not receive GH treatment during puberty had a lower bone mineral density than did GH-deficient patients who received GH replacement. The number of patients in the two groups was, however, small.

Several groups (Kaufman et al, 1992; Amato et al, 1993; O'Halloran et al, 1993; de Boer et al, 1994) have shown that reduced bone mineral density occurs in both isolated GH deficiency and in those with multiple pituitary hormone deficiencies. This suggests that the GH deficiency *per se*, rather than the under-treatment or over-treatment of additional pituitary hormone deficiencies, is causing the osteopenia.

Several of the studies in adults with childhood-onset GH deficiency have been short-term and provided different results depending on the design of the study, the dose of GH administered, the age of onset of GH deficiency in the study population and the technique used to measure bone mineral density. Some of the studies have shown no significant change in forearm cortical and integral bone mass (Binnerts et al, 1992; Degerblad et al, 1992;

Amato et al, 1993; Vandeweghe et al, 1993) and in lumbar spine integral bone mass (Vandeweghe et al, 1993) after 3–6 months GH replacement. However, Binnerts et al (1992) demonstrated a significant decrease in lumbar spine integral bone mineral density after 3 and 6 months of GH replacement. In contrast, we showed a significant increase in vertebral trabecular bone mineral density, measured by single-energy QCT, after 6 and 12 months, and a significant increase in forearm cortical and integral bone mineral content, measured using SPA, after 12 months of GH replacement in adults with childhood-onset isolated GH deficiency (O'Halloran et al, 1993). These findings illustrate that the response of bone mass to GH replacement depends on the type of bone being measured. A long-term study in adults with childhood-onset GH deficiency has shown a progressive increase in forearm cortical bone mineral content, lumbar spine integral bone mineral content and bone mineral density after 6–18 months of GH replacement. The most significant increase from base-line occurred 18 months after GH replacement (Vandeweghe et al, 1993).

Studies of biochemical markers of bone turnover have indicated that GH deficiency may be associated with decreased bone remodelling. Evidence for this comes from reduced serum levels of osteocalcin, a marker of bone formation, which have been demonstrated in children with GH deficiency (Johansen et al, 1990). Studies in adults with GH deficiency have produced contentious results, with either reduced (Sartorio et al, 1991; Amato et al, 1993) or normal osteocalcin levels (Johansen et al, 1990). GH stimulates bone turnover, with a significant increase in serum osteocalcin levels occurring in GH-deficient children (Johansen et al, 1990) receiving GH replacement.

Children with GH deficiency are reported to have a significant reduction in serum bone alkaline phosphatase concentration compared with control subjects (Sartorio et al, 1993a). In adult GH-deficient subjects, GH replacement has been shown to result in an increase in serum bone alkaline phosphatase concentration (Brixen et al, 1990; Sartorio et al, 1993b; Juul et al, 1994).

Sartorio et al (1993a) also demonstrated a significant reduction in serum ICTP, a marker of bone resorption, in children with GH deficiency, compared with healthy age-matched control subjects. Subsequently, an increase in serum ICTP concentration in adults with childhood-onset GH deficiency receiving GH replacement was demonstrated (Sartorio et al, 1993b).

The role of GH in the acquisition of bone mass also raises important issues concerning GH replacement in children with GH deficiency. At the present time, GH is discontinued on attainment of final height. It is becoming increasingly evident that this may be an inappropriate end-point and that attainment of peak bone mass may be a more important milestone.

SEX STEROIDS

The importance of sex steroids in the acquisition of bone mass is illustrated by young men with idiopathic hypogonadotrophic hypogonadism who have reduced bone mass before closure of the epiphyses has occurred, suggesting a defect in the acquisition of bone mass (Finkelstein et al, 1987). Other causes of hypogonadism in men associated with reduced bone mass include hyperprolactinaemia (Greenspan et al, 1986), Klinefelter's syndrome (Horowitz et al, 1992) and mild hypogonadism following chemotherapy for the treatment of Hodgkin's disease (Holmes et al, 1994). Hypogonadism in men appears to increase loss of both cortical and trabecular bone (Finkelstein et al, 1987).

Not only is exposure to increased levels of sex steroids important in the attainment of peak bone mass, but also the timing of such exposure appears to be critical. Young men in their early 20s with a history of untreated constitutional delay in growth and puberty (CDGP) (Finkelstein et al, 1992) show reduced cortical and trabecular bone mass, suggesting that the relative androgen deficiency at a critical stage in their development affected the acquisition of peak bone mass. Confirmatory evidence to support this interpretation would be provided if it could be shown that young men with CDGP who had previously received androgen therapy to advance the timing of their pubertal development had normal bone mineral density later in life. Such studies have not been published.

Dhuper et al (1990) studied bone mass of adolescent girls and related it to a score of integrated oestrogen exposure based on physiological events known to reflect circulating oestrogen levels. The subjects studied were selected to reflect a wide variation in the degree of oestrogen exposure. They found that those girls with the lowest oestrogen exposure during the pubertal years had the lowest cortical and integral bone mass.

Adult women with ovarian failure develop osteopenia. Bone mass is reduced after the menopause (Riggs and Melton, 1986), following bilateral oophorectomy (Richelson et al, 1984), in women with hyperprolactinaemic amenorrhoea (Klibanski et al, 1980; Biller et al, 1992), in amenorrhoeic athletes (Drinkwater et al, 1984) and in women with premature ovarian failure following chemotherapy for treatment of Hodgkin's disease (Redman et al, 1988; Kreuser et al, 1992). Osteopenia occurring shortly after the menopause is generally associated with a disproportionate loss of trabecular bone, whereas osteopenia occurring in older groups is more usually associated with proportionate loss of both cortical and trabecular bone (Riggs and Melton, 1983).

In men, oestrogen also plays a major role in bone mineralization and maturation. This was demonstrated in a 28-year-old adult male shown to have a disruptive mutation of the oestrogen receptor gene (Smith et al, 1994). This defect resulted in oestrogen resistance associated with high levels of serum oestradiol and oestrone. The administration of oral oestrogen, which was able to raise free serum oestradiol 10-fold, did not induce an increase in any oestrogen-dependent proteins (sex hormone-binding globulin, thyroxine-binding globulin, cortisol-binding globulin and prolactin) or change the levels of serum follicle-stimulating hormone (FSH) and luteinizing hormone (LH), which remained elevated. The bone mineral density of the lumbar spine was 3 standard deviations below the mean for age-matched normal women. There was biochemical evidence of increased bone turnover.

Serum androgen levels were normal and, despite progressing through puberty normally, there was incomplete epiphyseal closure, delayed skeletal maturation and osteopenia. This single patient with a specific gene defect demonstrates the importance of oestrogen for bone maturation and mineralization in men as well as in women.

Anorexia nervosa, although not a common problem in puberty, has an adverse effect on skeletal health. Reduced body mass itself contributes to reduced skeletal mass. Lack of oestrogen due to severely reduced gonadotrophin secretion will result in reduced bone mineral density. In addition, general malnutrition results in poor calcium intake as well as reduced body mass.

The management of osteopenia in these patients remains controversial. Regaining of weight is essential and has been shown to increase bone mass (Bachrach et al, 1991). Adequate calcium intake should also be ensured. In those who have not completed puberty, the use of oestrogen replacement requires fine judgement on an individual basis, as smaller doses of oestrogen stimulate growth but larger doses may compromise final height. In older patients, the replacement of oestrogen has been shown to prevent loss of the lumbar spine bone mass but not overall bone mass loss (Seeman et al, 1992).

In young adult women, secondary amenorrhoea from any cause for as little as 6 months may be associated with a significant reduction in bone mineral density (Davies et al, 1990).

In post-menopausal women, a decrease in femoral neck bone mineral density by 1 standard deviation from the age-adjusted mean increases the risk of hip fracture by a factor of 2.6 (Cummings et al, 1993). Post-menopausal oestrogen therapy prevents bone loss (Linsay et al, 1976; Stevenson et al, 1990; Ryde et al, 1994) and reduces the incidence of bone fracture (Hutchinson et al, 1979). Oral oestrogen (Linsay et al, 1976), trans-dermal oestrogen (Stevenson et al, 1990) and oestrogen implants (Ryde et al, 1994) are all effective in preserving bone mass in post-menopausal women.

In men with hyperprolactinaemic hypogonadism, restoration of normal testicular function is associated with a significant increase in cortical bone mass (Greenspan et al, 1986). Similarly, restoration of normal serum testosterone in men with idiopathic hypogonadotrophic hypogonadism is associated with a significant increase in cortical bone mass (Finkelstein et al, 1989).

INTERACTION OF SEX STEROIDS AND GH

The importance of both GH and sex steroids in the attainment of bone mass is of relevance when considering the treatment of children who have a combination of GH deficiency and either precocious puberty (Ogilvy-Stuart et al, 1994) or gonadotrophin deficiency. The current medical approach for the former combination is to prevent pubertal progression using a gonadotrophin-releasing hormone agonist while the child continues on GH replacement to maximize height before puberty is allowed to progress spontaneously. As acquisition of bone mass is influenced by the presence of sex steroids during the pubertal years, halting progression through puberty may have a deleterious effect on bone mass. Similarly, the timing of the introduction of sex steroid therapy in the GH-treated child with GH and gonadotrophin deficiencies may affect peak bone mass critically. In both situations, there is a fine balance between the requirement for further growth, the need for virilization/feminization and the acquisition of peak bone mass. It is not known whether GH therapy can compensate for the absence of sex steroids at this critical stage of development, although data derived from studies of bone mass in the female monkey suggest that this may be the case. In the animal study, GH treatment preserved peak bone mass in female monkeys who were made hypogonadal by the administration of a gonadotrophin-releasing hormone agonist (Mann et al, 1992).

TURNER'S SYNDROME

The most studied group of young patients with oestrogen deficiency is those with Turner syndrome and ovarian failure secondary to ovarian dysgenesis. Typically, these girls are oestrogen deficient throughout the whole of childhood from the earliest years. Therefore it might be expected that, in young adult life, girls with Turner syndrome would be osteopenic, although the exact contribution of the timing of oestrogen deficiency (early versus late childhood) is unclear. A number of studies have concluded that girls with Turner syndrome have reduced bone mineral density (Barr, 1974; Brown et al, 1978; Smith et al, 1982; Shore et al, 1982; Naeraa et al, 1991). As indicated earlier, however, there are problems in determining the significance of bone mineral density estimations in growing children, particularly, as in the case of Turner syndrome, where there is an additional pathological growth problem (skeletal dysplasia). Shore et al (1982) demonstrated that the mean radial bone mineral content of girls with Turner syndrome was 25.4% lower than that predicted by normalization for age, sex, height, weight and bone width using SPA. A quarter of this bone demineralization could be accounted for by delayed skeletal maturation. Some of the girls in this study were on oestrogen replacement, and although mineralization in this group was greater than in the group who received no oestrogen, it was still less than that seen in normal individuals. Patient selection by Shore et al (1982), however, may have affected the results, as some of the patients had been on GH replacement or oestrogen replacement, whereas others were untreated. In another report (Ross et al, 1991), girls with Turner syndrome aged 4–13, who had not received either long-term GH or oestrogen replacement were studied. When corrected for height and age, this group of patients had normal bone mineralization of the spine.

The question of bone mineral density in girls with Turner syndrome is important as some authorities justify the exposure of these patients to low doses of oestrogen during the pre-pubertal years as a means of improving final peak bone mass. There is, however, no evidence to support this approach. More recently, the situation has become complicated by the use of pharmacological doses of GH in the treatment of the statural problem associated with Turner syndrome. Neely et al (1993) evaluated girls with Turner syndrome who had received GH therapy but not oestrogen. Bone mineral content was reduced compared with normal age-matched control subjects. Mean bone mineral density, however, was not significantly reduced. Neely et al (1993) assessed bone mineral density using dual photon absorptiometry. After having adjusted bone mineral density for bone volume, they demonstrated that the mean bone mineral 'apparent' density of the spine and whole body was actually increased once chrono-logical age, bone age, height and pubertal stage had been taken into account. This study (Neely et al, 1993) fails to resolve the issue of whether or not the absence of oestrogen during early and mid-childhood com-promises the acquisition of a healthy skeleton in girls with Turner syndrome. It does, however, suggest that if they receive GH therapy, bone mineral density is normal. At present, the exposure of young girls with Turner syndrome to low doses of oestrogen in early childhood cannot be justified on the available evidence.

SUMMARY

Osteoporosis results from accelerated bone loss occurring after mid-life. The greater the bone mass accretion and bone mineralization in puberty and early adulthood, the less likely an individual is to develop clinically signifi-cant osteoporosis in later life.

The skeletal changes that occur in puberty are principally due to GH and sex steroids. As a consequence, any process that interferes with the normal physiology of these hormones during puberty, when the majority of peak bone mass accumulation and bone mineralization occurs, will have long-term implications for the development of osteoporosis. The main endocrine conditions of childhood influencing peak bone mass are GH deficiency, delayed puberty, gonadotrophin deficiency, Turner syndrome and male hypogonadism. Peak bone mass and bone mineralization are, however, also influenced by several other factors. These include genetic factors, particu-larly racial origin, and non-heritable variables, including body mass, adequate calcium intake during growth and physical activity. Therefore, chronic illnesses, malnutrition and anorexia nervosa will reduce bone mass. Appropriate management of these childhood conditions will decrease the risk of osteoporosis in adulthood.

REFERENCES

Albertsson-Wikland K, Roseberg S, Karlberg J et al (1994) Analysis of 24-hour growth hormone profiles of healthy boys and girls of normal stature: relation to puberty. *Journal of Clinical Endocrinology and Metabolism* **78:** 1195–1201.

Amato A, Carella C, Fazio F et al (1993) Body composition, bone metabolism and heart structure and function in growth hormone deficient adult before and after GH replacement therapy at low doses. *Journal of Clinical Endocrinology and Metabolism* **77**: 1671–1676.

Bachrach LK, Katzman DK, Litt IF et al (1991) Recovery from osteopenia in adolescent girls with anorexia nervosa. *Journal of Clinical Endocrinology and Metabolism* **72**: 602–606.

Barr DGO (1974) Bone deficiency in Turner's syndrome measured by metacarpal dimensions. *Archives of Diseases in Childhood* **49**: 821–822.

Biller BMK, Baum HBA, Rosenthal DI et al (1992) Progressive trabecular osteopenia in women with hyperprolactinaemic amenorrhoea. *Journal of Clinical Endocrinology and Metabolism* **75**: 692–697.

Binnerts A, Swart GR, Wilson JHP et al (1992) The effect of growth hormone administration in growth hormone deficient adults on bone, protein, carbohydrate and lipid homeostasis, as well as on body composition. *Clinical Endocrinology* **37**: 79–87.

Blumsohn A, Hannon RA, Wrate R et al (1994) Biochemical markers of bone turnover in girls during puberty. *Clinical Endocrinology* **40**: 663–670.

de Boer H, Blok GJ, Van Lingen AV et al (1994) Consequences of childhood-onset growth hormone deficiency for adult bone mass. *Journal of Bone and Mineral Research* **9**: 1319–1326.

Bonjour JP, Thientz G, Buchs B et al (1991) Critical years and stages of puberty for spinal and femoral bone mass accumulation during adolescence. *Journal of Clinical Endocrinology and Metabolism* **73**: 555–563.

Bonjour JP, Thientz G, Law F et al (1994) Peak bone mass. *Osteoporosis International* **15 (supplement 1):** 7–13.

Bourguignon JP, Vandeweghe M, Vanderschueren-Lodeweyckx M et al (1986) Pubertal growth and final height in hypopituitary boys: a minor role of bone age at onset of puberty. *Journal of Clinical Endocrinology and Metabolism* **63**: 376–382.

Brixen K, Nielsen HK, Mosekilde L & Flyvbjerg A (1990) A short course of recombinant human growth hormone treatment stimulates osteoblasts and activates bone remodeling in normal human volunteers. *Journal of Bone Mineral Research* **5**: 609–618.

Brown DM, Jowey J & Bradford DS (1978) Osteoporosis in ovarian dysgenesis. *Journal of Pediatrics* **84**: 816–820.

Corpas E, Harman SM, Pineyro MA et al (1992) Growth hormone-releasing hormone-(1–29) twice daily reverses the decreased GH and insulin-like growth factor-1 levels in old men. *Journal of Clinical Endocrinology and Metabolism* **75**: 530–535.

Cummings SR, Black DM, Nevitt MC et al (1993) Bone density at various sites for prediction of hip fractures. *Lancet* **341**: 72–75.

Davies MC, Hall ML & Jacobs HS (1990) Bone mineral loss in young women with amenorrhoea. *British Medical Journal* **301**: 790–793.

Degerblad M, Elgindy N, Hall K et al (1992) Potent effect of recombinant growth hormone on bone mineral density and body composition in adults with panhypopituitarism. *Acta Endocrinologica* **126**: 387–393.

Dhuper S, Warren MP, Brooks-Gunn J & Fox R (1990) Effects of hormonal status on bone density in adolescent girls. *Journal of Clinical Endocrinology and Metabolism* **71**: 1083–1088.

Drinkwater BL, Nilson K, Chesnut CH III et al (1984) Bone mineral content of amenorrheic and eumenorrheic athletes. *New England Journal of Medicine* **311**: 277–281.

Eriksen EF, Brixen K & Charles P (1995) New markers of bone metabolism: clinical use in metabolic bone disease. *European Journal of Endocrinology* **132**: 251–263.

Finkelstein JS, Klibanski A, Neer RM et al (1987) Osteoporosis in men with idiopathic hypogonadotrophic hypogonadism. *Annual of Internal Medicine* **106**: 354–361.

Finkelstein JS, Klibanski A, Neer RM et al (1989) Increases in bone density during treatment of men with idiopathic hypogonadotrophic hypogonadism. *Journal of Clinical Endocrinology and Metabolism* **69**: 776–783.

Finkelstein JS, Neer RM, Biller et al (1992) Osteopenia in men with a history of delayed puberty. *New England Journal of Medicine* **326**: 600–604.

Foresta C, Busnardo B, Ruzza et al (1983a) Lower calcitonin levels in young hypogonadic men with osteoporosis. *Hormone Metabolism and Research* **15**: 206–207.

Foresta C, Ruzza G, Mioni R et al (1983b) Testosterone and bone loss in Klinefelter syndrome. *Hormone Metabolism and Research* **15**: 56–57.

Gilsanz V, Gibbens DT, Roe TF et al (1988) Vertebral bone density in children: effect of puberty. *Radiology* **166**: 847–850.

Glastre C, Braillon P, David L et al (1990) Measurement of bone mineral content of the lumbar spine by dual energy x-ray absorptiometry in normal children: correlations with growth parameters. *Journal of Clinical Endocrinology and Metabolism* **70**: 1330–1333.

Greenspan SL, Neer RM, Ridgway EC & Klibanski A (1986) Osteoporosis in men with hyperprolactinaemic hypogonadism. *Annals of Internal Medicine* **104**: 777–782.

Ho KY, Evans WS, Blizzard RM et al (1987) Effects of sex and age on the 24-hour profile of growth hormone secretion in man: importance of endogenous estradiol concentrations. *Journal of Clinical Endocrinology and Metabolism* **64**: 51–58.

Holmes SJ, Whitehouse ST, Clark ST et al (1994) Reduced bone mineral density in men following chemotherapy for Hodgkin's Disease. *British Journal of Cancer* **70**: 371–375.

Horowitz M, Wishart JM, O'Loughlin PD et al (1992) Osteoporosis and Klinefelter's syndrome. *Clinical Endocrinology* **36**: 113–118.

Hutchinson TA, Polansky SM & Feinstein AR (1979) Post-menopausal oestrogens protect against fractures of hip and distal radius. *Lancet* **ii**: 705–709.

Hyer SL, Rodin DA, Tobias JH et al (1992) Growth hormone deficiency during puberty reduces adult bone mineral density. *Archives of Disease in Childhood* **67**: 1472–1474.

Inzucchi SE & Robbins RJ (1994) Clinical review 61: Effects of growth hormone on human bone biology. *Journal of Clinical Endocrinology and Metabolism* **79**: 691–694.

Iranmanesh A, Lizarralde G & Veldhuis JD (1991) Age and relative adiposity are specific negative determinants of the frequency and amplitude of growth hormone (GH) secretory bursts and the half-life of endogenous GH in healthy men. *Journal of Clinical Endocrinology and Metabolism* **73**: 1081–1088.

Johansen JS, Pedersen SA, Jorgensen JO et al (1990) Effects of growth hormone (GH) on plasma bone Gla protein in GH-deficient adults. *Journal of Clinical Endocrinology and Metabolism* **70**: 916–919.

Johnston CC Jr, Miller JZ, Slemenda CW et al (1992) Calcium supplementation and increases in bone mineral density in children. *New England Journal of Medicine* **327**: 82–87.

Juul A, Pedersen SA, Sørensen S et al (1994) Growth hormone treatment increases serum insulin-like growth factor binding protein-3, bone isoenzyme alkaline phosphatase and forearm bone mineral content in young adults with GH deficiency of childhood onset. *European Journal of Endocrinology* **131**: 41–49.

Katzman DK, Bachrach LK, Carter DR & Marcus R (1991) Clinical and anthropometric correlates of bone mineral acquisition in healthy adolescent girls. *Journal of Clinical Endocrinology and Metabolism* **73**: 1332–1339.

Kaufman JM, Taelman P, Vermeulen A & Vandeweghe M (1992) Bone mineral status in growth hormone deficient males with isolated and multiple pituitary deficiencies of childhood onset. *Journal of Clinical Endocrinology and Metabolism* **74**: 118–123.

Klibanski A, Neer RM, Beitins IZ et al (1980) Decreased bone density in hyperprolactinaemic women. *New England Journal of Medicine* **303**: 1511–1514.

Kreuser ED, Felsenberg D, Behles C et al (1992) Long-term gonadal dysfunction and its impact on bone mineralization in patients following COPP/ABVD chemotherapy for Hodgkin's disease. *Annals of Oncology* **3 (supplement 4)**: 105–110.

Linsay R, Hart DM, Aitken JM et al (1976) Long-term prevention of post-menopausal osteoporosis by oestrogen. *Lancet* **i**: 1038–1041.

Liu L, Merriam GR & Sherins RJ (1987) Chronic sex steroid exposure increases mean plasma growth hormone concentration and pulse amplitude in men with isolated hypogonadotrophic hypogonadism. *Journal of Clinical Endocrinology and Metabolism* **64**: 651–656.

Lloyd T, Andon MB, Rollings N et al (1993) Calcium supplementation and bone mineral density in adolescent girls. *Journal of the American Medical Association* **270**: 841–844.

Mann DR, Rudman CG, Akinbami MA & Gould KA (1992) Preservation of bone mass in hypogonadal female monkeys with recombinant human growth hormone administration. *Journal of Clinical Endocrinology and Metabolism* **74**: 1263–1269.

Martha PM & Reiter ED (1991) Pubertal growth and growth hormone secretion. *Endocrinology and Metabolism Clinics of North America* **20**: 165–182.

Mason HD, Martikainen H, Beard RW et al (1990) Direct gonadotrophic effect of growth hormone on oestradiol production by human granulosa cells in vitro. *Journal of Endocrinology* **126**: R1–R4.

Matkovic V & Heaney RP (1992) Calcium balance during human growth: evidence for a threshold behaviour. *American Journal of Clinical Nutrition* **55**: 992–996.

Naeraa RW, Brixen K, Hansen RM et al (1991) Skeletal size and bone mineral content in Turner's syndrome: relation to karyotype, oestrogen treatment, physical fitness, and bone turnover. *Calcification Tissue International* **49**: 77–83.

Neely EK, Marcus R, Rosenfeld RG & Bachrach LK (1993) Turner syndrome adolescents receiving growth hormone are not osteopenic. *Journal of Clinical Endocrinology and Metabolism* **76**: 861–866.

Ogilvy-Stuart AL, Clayton PE & Shalet SM (1994) Cranial irradiation and early puberty. *Journal of Clinical Endocrinology and Metabolism* **78**: 1282–1286.

O'Halloran DJ, Tsatsoulis A, Whitehouse RW et al (1993) Increased bone mineral density after recombinant human growth hormone therapy in adults with isolated GH deficiency. *Journal of Clinical Endocrinology and Metabolism* **76**: 1344–1348.

Patel DN, Pettifor JM & Becker PJ (1993) The effect of ethnicity on appendicular bone mass in white, coloured and Indian schoolchildren. *South African Medical Journal* **83(11)**: 847–853.

Politzer WS and Anderson JJB (1989) Ethnic and genetic differences in bone mass: a review with a hereditary vs environmental perspective. *American Journal of Clinical Nutrition* **50**: 1244–1259.

Redman JR, Bajorunas DR, Wong G et al (1988) Bone mineralisation in women following successful treatment of Hodgkin's disease. *American Journal of Medicine* **85**: 65–72.

Richelson LS, Wahner HW, Melton LJ III & Riggs BL (1984) Relative contributions of ageing and oestrogen deficiency to postmenopausal bone loss. *New England Journal of Medicine* **311**: 1273–1686.

Riggs BL & Melton LJ III (1983) Evidence for two distinct syndromes of involutional osteoporosis. *American Journal of Medicine* **75**: 899–891.

Riggs BL & Melton LJ III (1986) Involutional osteoporosis. *American Journal of Medicine* **314**: 1676–1686.

Rosenfield RL & Furlanetto R (1985) Physiologic testosterone or estradiol induction of puberty increases plasma somatomedin-C. *Journal of Pediatrics* **107**: 415–417.

Rosenfeld RG, Rosenbloom AL & Guevara-Aguirre J (1994) Growth hormone (GH) insensitivity due to primary GH receptor deficiency. *Endocrine Review* **15**: 369–390.

Ross JL, Long LM, Feuillan P et al (1991) Normal bone mineral density of the wrist and spine and increased wrist fractures in girls with Turner's syndrome. *Journal of Clinical Endocrinology and Metabolism* **73**: 355–369.

Ryde SJS, Bowen-Simpkins K, Bowen-Simpkins P et al (1994) The effect of oestradiol implants on regional and total bone mass: a three-year longitudinal study. *Clinical Endocrinology* **40**: 33–38.

Saggese G, Baroncelli GI, Bertelloni S et al (1993) Effects of long-term treatment with growth hormone on bone and mineral metabolism in children with growth hormone deficiency. *Journal of Pediatrics* **122**: 37–45.

Sartorio A, Conti A & Monzani M (1993a) New markers of bone and collagen turnover in children and adults with GH deficiency. *Postgraduate Medical Journal* **69**: 846–850.

Sartorio A, Conti A, Guzzaloni G & Faglia G (1991) Serum osteocalcin levels in patients with GH deficiency before and during GH treatment. *Acta Paediatrica Scandanavica* **80**: 100–102.

Sartorio A, Conti A, Monzani M et al (1993b) Growth hormone treatment in adults with GH deficiency: effects on new biochemical markers of bone and collagen turnover. *Journal of Endocrinology Investigations* **16**: 893–898.

Seeman E, Szmukler GI, Formica C et al (1992) Osteoporosis in anorexia nervosa: the influence of peak bone density, bone loss, oral contraceptive use, and exercise. *Journal of Bone and Mineral Research* **12**: 1467–1474.

Shore RM, Chesney RW, Mazess RB et al (1980) Bone mineral status in growth hormone deficiency. *Journal of Pediatrics* **96**: 393–396.

Shore RM, Chesney RW, Mazess RB et al (1982) Skeletal demineralisation in Turner's syndrome. *Calcification Tissue International* **34**: 519–522.

Smith EP, Boyd J, Frank GR et al (1994) Estrogen resistance caused by a mutation in the estrogen-receptor gene in a man. *New England Journal of Medicine* **331**: 1056–1061.

Smith MA, Wilson J & Price WH (1982) Bone demineralisation in patients with Turner's syndrome. *Journal of Medical Genetics* **19**: 100–103.

Stanhope R, Uruena M, Hindmarsh P et al (1991) Management of growth hormone deficiency through puberty. *Acta Paediatrica Scandinavica* **372** (**supplement**): 47–52.

Stevenson JC, Cust MP, Ganger KF et al (1990) Effects of transdermal versus oral hormone replacement therapy on bone density in spine and proximal femur in postmenopausal women. *Lancet* **336**: 265–269.

Theintz G, Buchs B & Rizzoli R (1992) Longitudinal monitoring of bone mass accumulation in healthy adolescents: evidence for a marked reduction after 16 years of age at the levels of lumbar spine and femoral neck in female subjects. *Journal of Clinical Endocrinology and Metabolism* **75:** 1060–1065.
Vandeweghe M, Taelman P & Kaufman JM (1993) Short and long-term effects of growth hormone treatment on bone turnover and bone mineral content in adult growth hormone deficient males. *Clinical Endocrinology* **39:** 409–415.
Young D, Hopper JL, Nowson CA et al (1995) Determinants of bone mass in 10 year old to 26 year old females—a twin study. *Journal of Bone and Mineral Research* **10:** 558–567.
Zamboni G, Antoniazzi F, Radetti G et al (1991) Effects of two different regimens of recombinant human growth hormone therapy on the bone mineral density of patients with growth hormone deficiency. *Journal of Pediatrics* **119:** 483–485.

Index

Note: Page numbers of article titles are in **bold** type.

365